The
Body Mind Connection
in
Human Movement Analysis

Edited by Susan Loman, M. A., ADTR
with
Rose Brandt, M.A.

With Foreword by
Martha Davis, Ph.D.

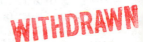
Published by
Antioch New England Graduate School
103 Roxbury Street
Keene, NH

TABLE OF CONTENTS

Acknowledgements   vii
Foreword   ix
     Martha Davis, Ph.D.
Preface   xv

**Part I: The KMP Perspective on Human
    Movement Analysis**

Clinical Applications of the KMP   21
     Susan Loman, M.A., A.D.T.R.
     K. Mark Sossin, Ph.D.

The Use of Expressive Arts in Prevention: 55
    Facilitating the Construction of Objects
     Judith S. Kestenberg, M.D.

Fetal Movement Notation: A Method of Attuning   93
to the Fetus
     Susan Loman, M.A., A.D.T.R.

Movement Retraining   109
     Arnhilt Buelte

**Part II: Expanding and Bridging
    the KMP Perspective**

Nonverbal Communication of Affect in Bali: 121
Movement in Parenting and Dance
     Janet Kestenberg-Amighi, Ph.D.
     Islene Pinder
     Judith Kestenberg, M.D.

The Essence of Gender in Movement   135
     Warren Lamb

Body Movement and Cognitive Style: 153
Validation of Action Profiling
     Deborah Du Nann Winter, Ph.D.

Body-Mind Dancing   203
     Martha Eddy, M.S., CMA

ACKNOWLEDGEMENTS

We deeply thank each of this volume's contributors: Janet Kestenberg-Amighi, Ph.D., Arnhilt Buelte, Martha Davis, Ph.D., Martha Eddy, M.S., CMA, Judith S. Kestenberg, M.D., Warren Lamb, Islene Pinder, K. Mark Sossin, Ph.D., and Deborah Du Nann Winter, Ph.D.

◆

We also thank Anne Brownell, M.A., Nancy Jo Cardillo, M.Ed., ADTR, Ellen Goldman, CMA, Smadar Korn, B.S.C., Penny Lewis, Ph.D. ADTR, RDT, Catherine McCoubrey, MCAT, DTR, CMA, Hillary Merman, M.Ed., ADTR, CMA, and Sandy Muniz-Lieberman, M.M.T., ADTR for their participation in the Second Annual KMP Conference.

◆

Our appreciation also to the Antioch New England Graduate School students who helped during the conference, typed manuscripts, and researched publishing requirements:
Christina Thurston and Mary Fish.
Special thanks to Maia Meeron, who designed the book and cover and spent several months editing, proofreading, typing and retyping material for publication.

◆

In addition, we thank James H. Craiglow, Provost, Julia Halevy, Chair, Department of Applied Psychology, and Eleanor Falcon, Director of Public Relations/Publications, of the Antioch New England Graduate School, for their support and encouragement.

ACKNOWLEDGEMENTS

Foreword

This is the second volume of papers related to the Kestenberg Movement Profile (KMP) and its potential for research, clinical practice and education. This volume demonstrates how well Dr. Kestenberg has inspired the talented individuals who have studied with her. The possibilities for the distinctive Kestenbergian view of movement analysis seem endless. Two papers are included on Action Profiling, which is something of a cousin to the KMP. They indicate how the theoretical framework and systematic coding developed by Judith Kestenberg can inform related research in fascinating ways.

This is not an introduction to the text, which clearly stands for itself as a demonstration of the state of the art of KMP research and application. Instead, this is a discussion of an issue critical to projects as complex and serious as the KMP research. As one who has known Dr. Kestenberg and her work for thirty years, through reading, conferences and personal discussions, I would like to take a position between the text and those readers relatively unfamiliar with movement analysis. The key question for the future is whether such work can and will become accessible to those outside of the circle of researchers and students who are immersed in it.

The KMP involves a microanalytic method of observation. One has only to pick up a college textbook on nonverbal communication to appreciate how subtle and detailed KMP observations are, compared to the great majority of nonverbal studies. Many researchers focus on microanalytic studies of only one variable, such as eye contact, and measure it in very simple ways. Of course, a dimension such as eye contact can be extraordinarily complex: consider the possible variations in timing, duration, direction and quality of gaze during a five-minute interaction between two people. One can spend hours studying a few minutes of eye contact, even without attending to other intimately associated movements, such as facial expression, direction of head turn, and blinking pattern. Most eye contact research consists of raters judging the change in amount of a single variable along a scale from none to a great deal.

This discussion will be limited to studies that directly observe actual behavior; it will exclude research that involves qualitative judgments of behavior, such as "warm," "cold," "in greater rapport," etc., without analysis of the movement details that make up these impressions. Nonverbal research based on direct observations may be roughly arranged along a continuum from simple to complex coding:

Simple: grossly recording one or a few variables, i.e., judgments of amount during a brief period using relative terms. For example, reporting none, rare, some, frequent, or constant eye contact.

Moderately Simple: Defining the beginnings and endings of a few dimensions of nonverbal behavior and tallying them over a period of time. For example, counting the number of head nods, position shifts, body rubbing actions, and speech gesticulations over 30 minutes.

Moderately Complex: Recording exact changes in a limited number of qualities or characteristics of the movement itself. For example, recording changes in direction, timing, and body part articulation.

Complex: Recording exact changes in more than four or five formal characteristics of movement to about a half-second level of accuracy. For example, doing a Labanotation of a dance movement (Hutchinson, 1970), or a Movement Signature Analysis of a 30-second segment of speech gesticulating (Davis, 1991).

Extremely Complex: Recording exact changes in more than four or five aspects of movement to finer than a half-second. For example, KMP notations of tension-flow, shape-flow, and effort and shape qualities of movement.

As one moves up this scale of complexity, not only are more variables involved, but a shift occurs from asking "what" to asking "how." The units of change become so small and subtle that they require either special instrumentation (such as EMG recording) or extensive observation training (the KMP). The writers in this text often use descriptive observations that are identifiable to the reader in order to convey the subject. But it must be understood that some movement patterns contained in the KMP are actually based on recordings of changes occurring in less than 1/2 to 1/10 of a second. Only trained observers can do this.

Which comes to a basic question. Those of us who have sat next to Dr. Kestenberg or some of her senior researchers for a glimpse of what they see, have been able to get enough of a visual and kinesthetic sense of the patterns to convince us of their existence and their importance. The experience is very compelling, and intuitively one appreciates that Dr. Kestenberg is onto something so important that her movement research should profoundly influence developmental theory and psychoanalysis. At the same time, one shakes one's head and worries that if a colleague experienced in movement observation cannot see these patterns very easily, how will intelligent laypersons, who are not going to get direct experience with KMP experts, understand the work? How can the KMP expert counter arguments by serious readers that they read too much into the behavior, that they project their own movements onto the page, that they make this up?

It is crucial to overcome this problem, or the work will stay limited to a small circle of the initiated. While experts trained in KMP can bridge the perceptual distance with vivid descriptions that readers may relate to in a general way, this is not sufficient. The average person will ultimately get a distorted view of Kestenberg's discoveries, because they are not gross patterns of tension or release, such a fluent movement that becomes arrested after a second or two. The patterns are more micro and only accurate observation can do them justice. Accuracy in recording *and* reporting of microanalytic patterns is essential for sound development and application of KMP assessment and theory.

The classic way to confirm the reliability of an observation method is to have several observers separately code the same behaviors, and then to statistically analyze the degree of observer agreement. K. Mark Sossin (1987) has contributed the greatest evidence for the reliability of KMP observations. But the system is so complicated that adequate samples, and comprehensive assessment of all the parameters, are too expensive to obtain. There is simply no grant money available today for reliability studies on such comprehensive observation methods. Unfortunately, reliability assessments must be limited to the observations of specific projects that limit and tailor the coding to answer specific questions.

But the fact that comprehensive assessments of reliability cannot be funded these days does not mean that the patterns do not exist. KMP profilers will have to turn to methods that the intelligent layperson can understand: recordings aided by instrumentation. I agree with those at the 1991 Conference on Movement Analysis Systems (sponsored by the Laban/Bartenieff Institute of Movement Studies), who argued for adaptation of modern motion analyzing instrumentation to verify complex movement observations. If KMP notators could record the movements of a subject who is both being videotaped and connected to an EMG apparatus, the person's tension-flow recordings could be superimposed on the video of the movement parallel with the EMG recordings. This would show the viewer that they are sufficiently parallel to EMG changes to confirm that the KMP observer is not projecting their own movement patterns on the subject. The viewer would also appreciate how fine these observations are. Similarly, instrumentation for measuring weight, force and time changes in position shifts and large movements could substantiate the acuteness and accuracy of the KMP observations of effort and flow qualities.

Another concern could then be raised: if these patterns can be measured electrically, who needs the observers? But the fact is that machinery is useless without observation experts. Examination of differences between instrument measures and individual observations can only be done by observation experts. Furthermore, there are many contexts in which subjects cannot be wired to machines. A vast array of situations require study only by observers. Similarly, computer analysis and generation of video images of movement is limited. Not only is the computer dependent on the input of the observation expert, but the electronic recording system will necessarily be limited in comparison with the full complexity of the actual movement.

In any case, KMP observations can only be conveyed with good film or video examples that are repeated, embellished with graphics, and enhanced with narrative so that the intelligent layperson can see the patterns. Without this, one cannot make experiential sense of the KMP literature.

These recommendations are relevant to all research on nonverbal communication that goes beyond the simple level of observation, of course. But they are critical for Kestenberg and Laban-related research that deals with nuances of movement quality that are difficult to convey in words or photographs. Without advances in how we convey and corroborate these observations, this research will remain relatively obscure. Nonverbal communication research of the past 20 years is awash with simple observation studies that have generated trivial results. Occasionally, a simple analysis can be inspired and productive, but for the most part, complex observations are what demonstrate the full potential of the subject. The Kestenberg Movement Profile is one of the most promising of these efforts, and deserves widespread recognition and use. The challenge to Dr. Kestenberg and her associates is to exploit modern technology to make their observations and discoveries accessible to a wider audience.

Martha Davis, Ph.D.
Clinical Psychologist

References

Davis, M. (1991). Guide to Movement Analysis Methods: Part 1 Movement Signature Analysis, Part 2 Movement Psychodiagnostic Inventory, Part 3 Nonverbal Interaction and States Analysis. Unpublished manuscript.

Hutchinson, A. (1970). Labanotation. New York: Theatre Arts Books.

Sossin, K. M. (1987). Reliability of the Kestenberg Movement Profile. In Movement Studies, Vol. 2, pp. 23-28.

Preface

The concept for this book arose out of our Second Annual Kestenberg Movement Profile Conference entitled, *The Kestenberg Movement Profile: Research and Works in Progress.* As was the case after the First Conference, we were very inspired by the quality of the presentations and wished to preserve them by creating a volume of articles generated from the event.

Directly derived from the Conference are five ground-breaking pieces of work on new areas of application in the field. Judith Kestenberg, the originator of the KMP, expands the sphere of her profile into the arenas of visual art, dance and music in her contribution, *The Use of Expressive Arts in Prevention: Facilitating the Construction of Objects.* Of special interest are Kestenberg's descriptions of movement observable within the artwork of Renaissance masterpieces and in the drawings of children, representing all five phases of movement development depicted in the profile. Reproductions of the artwork, which illuminate and enliven the movement examples, are included in the paper.

Applying the KMP to various cultures has been of ongoing interest. The team of Kestenberg-Amighi, Pinder, and Kestenberg write about their work both in the field and in analyzing KMPs of children and adults in Bali, in *Nonverbal Communication of Affect in Bali: Movement in Parenting and Dance.*

As a practical application of the KMP with infants, toddlers and their parents, Arnhilt Buelte shares her vast experience as co-director for 18 years of the Center for Parents and Children in her article entitled, *Movement Retraining.* She clearly describes the sequential development of movement patterns from infancy through walking and provides ideas for movement interventions at various stages. Special attention is given to optimal positions for holding and supporting young children. Educators may find her descriptions useful in pinpointing sources of developmental difficulties in children.

Warren Lamb takes on the challenging task of searching for intrinsic gender differences in movement through his observations made in Europe, North America, Africa, India and Southeast Asia. *The Essence of Gender in Movement* offers the view that while transcending cultural conditioning, men and women still move differently.

Through clinical vignettes of our respective work as clinical psychologist and dance/movement therapist, Mark Sossin and I present aspects of the KMP which are useful in diagnosis and treatment planning in preventative and therapeutic settings. *Clinical Applications of the Kestenberg Movement Profile* includes examples of actual work with child and adult clients.

As the process of developing this book unfolded, our earlier objective, of simply documenting the conference, became too narrow. We wished to broaden the scope of the book and include research and works in progress on human movement analysis topics which would more generally appeal to those interested in the body-mind connection.

Fortunately, we learned that Deborah Du Nann Winter, an Action Profiler, was interested in sharing her research paper, *Body Movement and Cognitive Style: Validation of Action Profiling,* with us. Four experiments are reported in her contribution to answer the provocative question of whether the Action Profile might provide a useful method for studying motoric elements of human thought process.

To reach the dance world, we included Martha Eddy's inspirational dance form, which bridges the Kestenberg Movement Profile system with Laban Movement Analysis, Body-Mind Centering™ and spirituality. *Body-Mind Dancing*™ describes her dance form which integrates the artistic and the physiological processes of the body involving improvisation, vocalization, hands-on work and anatomical discussion, as well as movement sequences.

I also took the opportunity to include an article which I wrote on the application of the KMP to pregnancy since that particular approach to "preparation for the child" was so valuable to me as a first-time parent. *Fetal Movement Notation: A Method of Attuning to the Fetus* reviews ways that expectant parents can learn about aspects of their child's temperament by feeling and recording the baby's kicks, flutters and presses in utero.

Martha Davis, a prominent researcher and author in this field for the past 25 years and the originator of "Movement Signature Analysis" graciously agreed to write the foreword for this book. Her perspectives and insights are greatly appreciated as she is able to place the KMP and Laban-related systems in the context of current work in the field of nonverbal communication research.

Susan Loman, M.A., A.D.T.R., Editor

Part I:
The KMP Perspective on
Human Movement Analysis

Clinical Applications of the Kestenberg Movement Profile

K. Mark Sossin, Ph.D.
Susan Loman, M.A., A.D.T.R.

Introduction

The Kestenberg Movement Profile (KMP) is a complex instrument for describing, assessing and interpreting nonverbal behavior. It graphically depicts 120 distinct movement factors (across 29 polar dimensions) and includes descriptions of body attitudes and qualifying numerical data. These are derived and calculated from a notation system that has its roots in Laban Movement Analysis.

Dr. Judith Kestenberg, the originator of the KMP (1965a, 1965b, 1967, 1975; Kestenberg, Marcus, Robbins et. al., 1971; Kestenberg & Sossin, 1979), has made important clinical and theoretical contributions to psychoanalysis through the observation of infants, children and adults. The KMP was derived from Rudolph Laban's motion factors (1947, 1960), and influenced by Warren Lamb's (1965) interpretation of their use and structure (Ramsden, 1973). The interpretation system underlying the KMP is Anna Freud's developmental psychoanalytic metapsychology (1965).

Over many years, Judith Kestenberg has pursued an enduring inquiry into the nature and significance of nonverbal behavior. In the early 1950's, recognizing that her methodology was inadequate, she devoted extensive study to Effort/Shape Analysis with experts in movement and dance. By 1953, Dr. Kestenberg had begun longitudinal studies of the movement patterns of three children, who were each followed for 20 years. Then, nearly 30 years ago, Dr. Kestenberg's investigations into the role of nonverbal behavior in treatment and assessment were pursued further within the collaborative context of the Sands Point Movement Study Group (comprised of Dr.

Kestenberg, Dr. Hershey Marcus, Dr. Jay Berlowe, Dr. Esther Robins, Arnhilte Buelte and Martha Soodak). The group realized that little was known from a psychoanalytic perspective, and even less was standardized. Moreover, they were concerned not just with adults but also with pre-verbal infants and children and, ideally, sought a methodology that would apply comparable measures to the infant, child and adult.

Those applying the newly-evolving method notated infants on neonatal units, as well as children in nursery schools and well-baby clinics. As the Kestenberg Movement Profile emerged, children were observed and followed on kibbutzim. From 1972 through 1990, the Center for Parents and Children of Child Development Research was operated on Long Island, for the purpose of primary prevention. Research at the Center followed pregnant women and had the opportunity to follow children, along with their mothers and fathers, from birth through age four. In this context, the largest number of movement profiles were made — from live observation, film and video recordings — since periodic movement observations were a regular part of the ongoing assessment. This also provided opportunities to apply and clarify the diagnostic usage of the KMP in relation to clinically-known adults and children.

The KMP has evolved methodologically and interpretively during more than 30 years of research by Kestenberg and her colleagues. Their findings have linked the dominance of specific movement patterns with particular developmental phases and psychological functions. The KMP framework has been the basis of a wide range of psychoanalytically-oriented observational studies: obsessive-compulsive development (Kestenberg, 1966, 1980a), transitional objects and body-image formation (Kestenberg & Weinstein, 1978), organ-object and self- and object-representations (Kestenberg, 1971), bisexuality and activity/passivity (Kestenberg & Marcus, 1979), mother-infant holding and methods in infant and adult therapy (Kestenberg & Buelte, 1977a, 1977b, 1983; Kestenberg, 1985), paternal development (Kestenberg, Marcus, Sossin & Stevenson, 1982), and transitional phases in development (Kestenberg & Buelte, 1980). Movement observation has complemented Kestenberg's (1975, 1976,

1980b) investigations of female sexuality, pregnancy and maternal feelings, and of obsessive-compulsive disorder.

The dominant focus of much of this research has been the development of techniques for the primary prevention of emotional disorders. The KMP's specialized movement language, and its body of theory and research, can only be summarized in this paper, which draws primarily on the work of Kestenberg and Sossin (1979). The interested reader is referred to Laban, Lamb, Kestenberg (1965a, 1965b, 1967, 1975), Kestenberg, Marcus, Robbins et. al., (1971) and Bartenieff & Lewis (1980) for further relevant material, as well as a previous compilation in the current series (Lewis & Loman, 1990).

The KMP's information about intrapersonal psychological functioning is applicable to all age groups; some patterns may even be studied in the womb. Any two or more profiles (e.g., mother and child) can be compared with each other to yield information about areas of interpersonal conflict and harmony. At the Center for Parents and Children, the profile was used to assess the interpersonal dynamics among family members, as well as to evaluate congenital movement preferences, levels of developmental achievement, levels of fixation or regression, and factors indicative of cognitive abilities.

Students at Antioch New England Graduate School have begun to utilize the KMP in their master's theses (Bridges, 1989; Hastie-Atley, 1991; Lemon, 1990), but many areas of potentially fruitful research and clinical application have yet to be pursued. For example, the KMP could be applied as an ethnogrammatic tool of movement observation, outside of the psychoanalytic context. It could be amended for specific research purposes, such as anthropological investigations, or to focus on specific clinical populations; such applications lie ahead. Unlike rating scales, the KMP is a complex instrument, requiring skilled and experienced notators. Although professional interest in the KMP is growing, there are still relatively few trained KMP notators. No doubt the KMP's complexity has limited the quantity and breadth of its applications to date. The aim of this paper is to present some aspects of the KMP which are useful in diagnosis and

Figure 1. KMP of a 13-Month Old Boy
(Some statistics not included.)

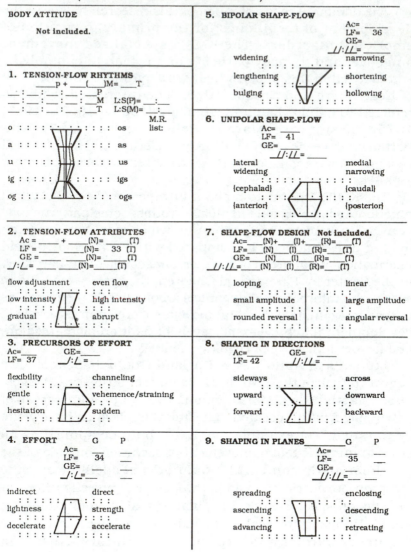

BODY ATTITUDE

Not included.

1. TENSION-FLOW RHYTHMS
___p + ___(___)M= ___ T
__ : __ : __ : __ : __ P
__ : __ : __ : __ : __ M   L:S(P)= __:__
__ : __ : __ : __ : __ T   L:S(M)= __:__
                                           M.R.
o : : : : . . . . : : : os   list:
a : : : : : : : : : as
u : : : : : : : : : us
ig : : : : : : : : : igs
og : : : : . : : : : ogs

2. TENSION-FLOW ATTRIBUTES
Ac = ___ + ___(N)= ___(T)
LF = ___ ___(N)= 33 (T)
GE = ___ ___(N)= ___(T)
$\diagup$:L = ___ ___(N)= ___(T)

flow adjustment   even flow
low intensity   high intensity
gradual   abrupt

3. PRECURSORS OF EFFORT
Ac=___   GE=___
LF= 37 $\diagup$:L = ___

flexibility   channeling
gentle   vehemence/straining
hesitation   sudden

4. EFFORT   G   P
Ac=   ___ ___
LF=   34   ___
GE=   ___ ___
$\diagup$:L=___ ___

indirect   direct
lightness   strength
decelerate   accelerate

5. BIPOLAR SHAPE-FLOW
                              Ac= ___
                              LF= 36
                              GE= ___
                              $\diagup/$:$\diagup\diagup$ = ___
widening   narrowing
lengthening   shortening
bulging   hollowing

6. UNIPOLAR SHAPE-FLOW
                  Ac= ___
                  LF= 41
                  GE= ___
                  $\diagup/$:$\diagup\diagup$ = ___
lateral   medial
widening   narrowing
{cephalad}   {caudal}
{anterior}   {posterior}

7. SHAPE-FLOW DESIGN   Not included.
Ac=___(N)+___(I)+___(R)=___(T)
LF=___(N)___(I)___(R)=___(T)
GE=___(N)___(I)___(R)=___(T)
$\diagup/$:$\diagup\diagup$=___(N)___(I)___(R)=___(T)

looping   linear
small amplitude   large amplitude
rounded reversal   angular reversal

8. SHAPING IN DIRECTIONS
Ac=___   GE= ___
LF= 42 $\diagup/$:$\diagup\diagup$ = ___

sideways   across
upward   downward
forward   backward

9. SHAPING IN PLANES___   G   P
                  Ac=   ___ ___
                  LF=   35   ___
                  GE=   ___ ___
                  $\diagup/$:$\diagup\diagup$=___ ___

spreading   enclosing
ascending   descending
advancing   retreating

treatment planning, with special emphasis on applications in dance/movement therapy. The authors will draw vignettes from their work with both children and adults, in preventative and therapeutic settings.

Summary of the KMP

Each of the nine KMP diagrams refers to a specific kind of movement pattern (Figure 1 is an example of a KMP profile). The observational, developmental and interpretive characteristics of the KMP's movement patterns are summarized below.

Tension-Flow Attributes

Tension-Flow is a manifestation of animate muscle elasticity. Bound flow is a restraining movement which occurs when agonist and antagonist muscles contract simultaneously. Free flow is a releasing movement which occurs when a contraction of the agonist muscles is not counteracted by the antagonists. Neutral flow refers to a range of flow changing continuously over time, varying the relative levels of bound flow and free flow.

Tension-flow can also be classified in terms of its attributes (or intensity factors), which describe tension changes along three dimensions:

- remaining **even** or **adjusting**;
- expressing **high** or **low intensity**;
- changing **abruptly** or **gradually**.

Tension-flow attributes are preferences for aggressive or indulging patterns of arousal and quiescence. These preferences are present from birth (and even before); they show increasing stability as the individual matures, influenced both by developmental factors and by individual temperament. Although tension-flow patterns continue throughout childhood and into adulthood, as needs and affects become subordinated to ego-based reality functioning, they tend to become subordinated to more advanced movement factors.

Interpretively, tension-flow is linked to affect regulation: bound flow and aggressive attributes are associated with cautious feelings, while free flow and indulging attributes are associated with carefree feelings. More subtle or complex affects are related to combinations of tension-flow attributes. Tension-flow regulation through the selection of tension-flow attributes is intrinsic to tension-flow rhythms.

Tension-Flow Rhythms

The KMP's view of development proceeds through a sequence of psychoanalytically and psychosexually conceived developmental phases, reflecting the tension-flow rhythms (see Kestenberg & Sossin, 1979). As development proceeds through each phase, preferences for different movement patterns surface and change and are reflected in the qualities of movement which are most likely to be used.

Variations between free and bound flow are rhythmic, although irregular, in their intervals. Ten rhythmic patterns have been identified, corresponding in pairs to the five major developmental phases: oral, anal, urethral, inner-genital and outer genital (Kestenberg, 1975). The ten basic rhythms are sucking, biting, twisting, straining, running, stopping/starting, undulating, swaying, jumping, and leaping. Although, for example, the oral/sucking rhythm is prototypic of the oral libidinal phase, all body parts can show all rhythms, and all rhythmic patterns are evident (to greater or lesser extents) at all phases. Frequency distributions appear to reflect consistent individual differences. Other body parts, such as the fingers or toes, may also show these rhythms, and the different areas of the body may express consistent or inconsistent rhythmic patterns. In addition to the ten basic rhythms, there is great variety of mixed rhythms, combinations of two or more rhythms. Individuals' preferences for specific tension-flow rhythms indicate their preferred methods of drive discharge. Comparison of tension-flow rhythm patterns in interpersonal relationships, such as between mother and child, reveals the areas of potential complementarity or conflict in the relationship, in terms of needs.

Precursors of Effort

Laban used the term effort (1960; Laban & Lawrence, 1947) to describe movement changes (including tension-flow) in relationship to space, weight and time. Efforts are developmentally preceeded by precursors of effort, affectively charged ways of manipulating the external environment, which become motor counterparts of defense mechanisms and styles of learning. The KMP uses six pairs of precursors of effort: **channeling** vs. **flexible**, **straining** vs. **gentle**, and **sudden** vs. **hesitating**. The first element of each pair is aggressive, while the second element is indulgent. For example, channeling keeps tension levels even to follow precise pathways; this has an aggressive character. Its opposite, the flexible precursor of effort, changes tension levels to move around in space, which implies avoidance (which may be put to defensive use) and is thus more indulgent. In terms of defense mechanisms, isolation can take the form of channeling, using an even flow of tension. Like defenses, the precursors of effort can be either problematic or constructive (isolation can be either affective disassociation or objective thinking). The precursors of effort are both body-oriented, in terms of tension-flow, and reality-oriented, in terms of space, weight and time; hence, they mediate between tension-flow and effort.

Effort

Efforts are the motor components of coping with external reality in terms of space, weight and time. In space, these are **directness** and **indirectness**; in weight, **strength** and **lightness**; and in time, **acceleration** and **deceleration**. Directness, strength and acceleration are aggressive effort elements, while indirectness, lightness and deceleration are more accommodating ways of dealing with space, weight and time. Each individual gradually develops their own characteristic distribution of effort elements. The line of development of an effort element may be traced back to a specific precursor of effort and, even further, to a specific tension-flow attribute pattern. The individual's mature constellation of effort elements shows their preferences in terms of attention, intention and decision-making.

Bipolar Shape-Flow

Changes in shape-flow express shifts in affective relations

with objects in the environment. Bipolar shape-flow is the symmetrical growing and shrinking of the body in response to environmental stimuli. In terms of breathing, for example, we grow with inhalation and shrink with exhalation. Growing and shrinking occur in three dimensions: horizontal (width), vertical (length) and sagittal (depth). Bipolar shape-flow expresses the individual's emotional response to the environment, and structures their discharge of aggressive and libidinal drives.

Unipolar Shape-Flow

In unipolar shape-flow, the body grows and shrinks asymmetrically, expressing attraction or repulsion toward discrete stimuli. Unipolar shape-flow also occurs in three dimensions: horizontal (lateral vs. medial), vertical (cephalad vs. caudal) and sagittal (anterior vs. posterior). In a vertical unipolar movement the body grows only upward or downward (vs. a vertical bipolar movement which lengthens both upward and downward). Unipolar shape-flow evolves from reflexive behavior and becomes a system of extending the body in space (shaping of space in directions).

Shape-Flow Design

Along with changes in body shape, body movement also creates designs in personal space. These movements can be either away from the body (centrifugal) or toward the body (centripetal). They are classified in terms of their linearity, their degree of amplitude and their angularity. Shape-flow design is notated somewhat like tension-flow, with synchronously drawn symbols for movement features. Shape-flow design patterns reflect the individual's style of relating and feelings of relatedness. They are influenced by cultural conditioning, congenital preferences, developmental stage and situational factors.

Shaping of Space in Directions

Shaping in directions is formed by the linear projection of the body into dimensional space. These directional movements bring distant objects into local space. Directions in space include moving **across** the body and moving **sideways** (horizontal), moving **downward** and moving **upward** (vertical), and moving **backward** and moving **forward** (sagittal). Directional patterns are associated with precursors of effort, defenses against external stimuli, and environmental learning responses. Closed-shape directions (moving sideways, upward and forward) form the outer limits of bodily access, creating new boundaries. For example, moving across the body creates a shield against frontal and side attack, while moving sideways eludes attacks from the back and side. Learned responses are linked to these defenses; for example, moving backwards, a defense against frontal attack, is associated with suddenness, allowing the mover to quickly avoid an aggressor.

Shaping in Space in Planes

Shaping in planes configures space by creating concave or convex shapes. Horizontal shaping **encloses** or **spreads**; vertical shaping **descends** or **ascends**; sagittal shaping **retreats** or **advances**. However, each spatial plane includes a principal and an accessory dimension. In the horizontal plane, the accessory dimension is sagittal; spreading and enclosing are used in exploration. In the vertical plane, the accessory dimension is horizontal; ascending and descending are used in confrontation. In the sagittal plane, the accessory dimension is vertical; advancing and retreating are used in anticipatory actions. Interpretively, shaping of space in planes expresses multi-dimensional relationships with objects and their internalized images.

The Two Systems

The tension-flow/effort system (System 1), shown by the diagrams on the left side of the KMP (Figure 1), depicts developmentally evolving patterns of dealing with internal and external reality. The shape-flow/shaping system (System 2), shown by the diagrams on the right side, depicts developmentally evolving patterns of spatial movement expressing growing complexity of object relations. The two systems resonate interpretively: aggressive tension-flow/effort patterns are affined (fit well), with shrinking shape-flow and closed shaping; pleasant and indulging tension-flow/effort patterns are affined with growing shape-flow and open shaping.

Other Integral Features of the KMP

The KMP is statistically constructed, and organized to optimize its use as a descriptive tool; however, it can only summarize the complex processes involved in human movement. The raw notational data supplements the profile, especially with the individual's characteristic patterns of phrasing, the uni-phasic or multi-phasic ordering of movement patterns. Certain patterns may appear more in the introduction, main theme, ending or transition of a phrase. Phrases can be analyzed for the stochastic processes (sequential contingencies) that they may show. Preferences for specific ways of combining patterns can also be detailed only by examining the raw data.

Movement can occur in gestures, using just one part of the body, or in postures, involving the entire body (Lamb, 1965, 1987; Ramsden 1973). Movement phrases sometimes show the same patterns, first in a gesture and then in a posture, or vice versa. These sequences are called gesture-posture or posture-gesture merging, and are generally not integrated until adolescence. Interpretively, postures indicate a wider range of intrapsychic elements than gestures, since they require greater bodily participation.

The dimensions of a KMP diagram reflect the relative weighting of its elements. Its overall size, however, is a function of the load factor, the composite of all inputs in a subsystem. The load factor shows the complexity of the subsystem, by indicating how many elements are involved in an action, between one (33% load factor) and three (100% load factor). It enables comparison of the relative complexity of each subsystem.

Another important statistic is the gain-expense ratio, which compares the number of movement attributes or elements (gain) per subsystem to the number of movement flow factors (expense) in notated phrases. The gain-expense ratio is interpreted in relation to other subsystems, and indicates the relative degree of affective control vs. affective spontaneity in each area. This affective component is further broken down into a ratio of free flow to bound flow (System 1) or a ratio of growing and shrinking per subsystem (System 2).

Flow Factors

From birth (or earlier), two basic modes of self-regulation are observable: we term them tension-flow and shape-flow. These modes correspond to two modes of action which are common to all living tissue, whether a cell, an organ, or an organism: elasticity and plasticity. To illustrate, we might picture a compressed spring: the tension-flow is bound and the shape-flow is shrinking; we release the spring, and we see it grow in free tension-flow.

Both tension-flow and shape-flow are fundamental in the experience and expression of affect. Bound flow corresponds to inhibition, discontinuity and to affects related to danger (anxiety), whereas free-flow corresponds to facilitation of impulses, continuity and to affects related to release and safety (Kestenberg & Buelte, 1983). In free flow, agonist muscles are not met with counteraction by antagonists (e.g., an easy-flowing, unrestrained fling of the hand); in bound flow, antagonist and agonist muscles co-contract together (e.g., the tightening of a fist).

Affined with Bound Flow ("Aggressive")	Affined with Free Flow ("Indulging")
even level	tension-flow adjustment
high intensity	low intensity
abrupt changes	gradual changes

Tension-Flow Attributes (TFAs) pertain to more specific feelings of pleasure and safety (ease) and of displeasure and danger (caution), and preferred patterns of an individual's temperament. We are likely to see more even flow in an individual who is indifferent or quite composed. Flow adjustment is more likely seen in flirtation or shyness. These patterns are also prerequisites for holding and shifting attention. We see increasing tension to high intensity in mounting excitement, anger and anxiety; we see decreasing tension to low intensity in calming, soothing and subsiding excitement. We abruptly change our tension level when we are startled, surprised or impatient. We gradually change our tension level when we are reposed, deliberate or patient.

Tension-flow attributes are not themselves affects, rather they are the medium of expression of affects of pleasure and displeasure. Shades and complexities of these affects are related to the varied combinations, sequences and intervals between changes that characterize the flow. For example, contrast an abruptly adopted stare, evenly held in high-intensity bound flow (as when stern or frightened) with a gradual easing of tension, mildly adjusting the brow (as when indulging in a pleasant thought) (Sossin, 1983; Kestenberg, 1985).

A patient may speak in a manner characterized by high intensity and abruptness; the clinician who responds to this client in low intensity and graduality will present a clashing, non-attuned pattern. Though each therapist brings his or her own temperament (and TFAs) to bear, it is intrinsic to the analytic process to speak to the patient with a reasonable degree of attunement; too great a breach of attunement will interfere with the patient's understanding of what the analyst has said. An upset child, who becomes highly intense, will not hear the clinician who is speaking in low intensity. Once the therapist attunes to him in high intensity, the child may follow the therapist into a less intense, calmer state.

The relative similarity or difference in TFA constellation is one measure of attunement; and moreover, it is one of at least three distinct types of affect attunement that can be measured using the KMP. In fact, attunement in tension-flow appears to be a key manifestation of empathy between parent and child. Therefore, there should be a high correlation between such measures of attunement and the ratings of clashing and a maternal sensitivity, as used in the attachment theory model.

Shape-Flow (Bipolar/Unipolar)

Our classification of patterns differentiates between three types of affective experience. As opposed to the pleasure and displeasure of tension-flow, attributes of shape-flow are expressive of comfort and discomfort (when changes are bipolar) and are also expressive of repulsion and attraction (when the changes are unipolar). Shape-flow is a manifestation of plasticity; its basic elements are the growing and shrinking of body shape. It shows interaction, especially affective relations, with stimuli and objects in the environment (i.e., Balint's "environmental objects"). Bipolar shape-flow is symmetric in pattern. The prototype of shape-flow is breathing: people grow as they inhale and shrink as they exhale, expanding and contracting, stretching and compressing, taking in and expelling. Growing and shrinking occur in three body dimensions: width/horizontal, length/vertical and depth/sagittal.

The expansion of growing in bipolar shape flow is the physical basis of primary narcissism. From the bipolar patterns, one can assess feelings of well-being, and the degree to which an individual requires narcissistic supplies. Ideally, the parent grows into the child as the child grows into the parent. In the absence of parental responsiveness and mutuality of interaction, the child may show an excessive growing out into the world, i.e., an excessive degree of narcissistic neediness. Physical illness often leads to bipolar shrinking (e.g., bipolar shortening in colic, bipolar narrowing in asthma, or bipolar hollowing in disorders involving regurgitation).

There is a developmental progression from bipolarity to unipolarity. In unipolar shape-flow, the growing and shrinking is asymmetrical — in response to more distinct stimuli (Kestenberg & Sossin, 1979; Sossin, 1983). If a noxious stimulus becomes localized on one's left side, then one might narrow (withdraw from it) with the left shoulder only. The child grows toward the mother who helps him or her. We speculate that unipolar shape-flow patterns evolve from spinal reflexes, and then become embedded into a system of extending bodily dimensions into the surrounding space.

To review, these three classifications of movement, tension-flow, bipolar shape-flow and unipolar shape-flow (and their attributes), distinguish affective responses of safety/danger, comfort/discomfort and attraction/repulsion. Moreover, within this formulation, plasticity gives structure to elasticity; and, affects arising in relationships structure other affective responses.

The KMP in Dance/Movement Therapy

Dance therapists have increasingly drawn upon psychodynamic developmental models in framing their clinical interventions (Siegel, 1974, 1984; Sandel, 1982; Lewis, 1984, 1986, 1990; Dosamantes, 1990). The KMP offers a developmental framework which can be used to encourage and measure growth, and to integrate progressive interventions with the developmental process. It describes the normal developmental process in movement terms, which aid in identifying deviations from the norm, as well as strengths and latent potentials. The KMP's psychodynamic framework provides information about drive development, affects, defenses against drives, defenses against objects, ego and superego functioning, object relations, narcissism, and areas of conflict or harmony in dynamics and object relationships.

The diagnostic/interpretive application of the KMP can lead to the detection of specific early developmental deficits and areas of psychic conflict, and suggests which movement patterns will be likely to foster resolution and growth. For example, the profile can indicate delayed, missed, distorted, or prematurely-induced developmental milestones by showing scanty or overabundant amounts of phase-appropriate movement patterns. Specific problems caused by trauma, such as abuse, separation or illness, during a specific phase of childhood, may affect the shape of diagrams in the KMP. When children experience these difficulties, they feel a sense of inadequacy which affects their self-image and often endures into later life. Body-image distortions, restrictions of movement, and accident-proneness may all be remnants of childhood trauma. The KMP identifies the specific movement patterns that are most relevant to the early conflicts between a specific caretaker and the child (such as inadequate holding and support or constitutional temperamental differences) that had, or are having, a formative impact upon the child's movement repertoire.

Once a deficit or problem area in movement patterning is recognized in the KMP, various channels of intervention can be explored. By offering a systematic way to discern an individual's movement repertoire, and to correlate it with psychological experience, the KMP offers a stratagem for approaching treatment. Dance/movement therapists often use tension-flow attunement to develop affective empathy, and shape-flow responsiveness to develop trust (Kestenberg & Buelte, 1977a). These processes can evolve into more mature movement interactions when the patient is ready.

Dance/movement therapists operate in many different professional settings, and the KMP provides them with a powerful tool to assess patients in developmental and psychodynamic terms. To optimally use the KMP, the therapist would evaluate the patient's progress with a complete pre-treatment and post-treatment profile. In treatment planning, the KMP would be used to identify strengths as well as deficits, guide the therapists' movement approaches, and help the therapist determine whether to use attunement, mirroring, or affined movement patterns with the patient (Loman, 1991).

Clinical Relevance of Developmental Transitions

In normal development, there is an alternating balance between stabilization and mobilization of body attitudes. Transitions from one body attitude to the next are accomplished with mobility and consolidated with stability (Kestenberg & Buelte, 1983).

The body's shape or alignment, the body attitude, progresses from a ball-like state (the fetus and newborn), to horizontal stretching (promoting rolling), to quadrupedal stability (leading to crawling on all fours), to vertical standing, and finally to sagittal balancing (leading to walking). The child mobilizes to produce these transitions in alignment by rolling over in the horizontal floor space, crawling on all fours, walking sideways, and walking forward.

This mobility requires phase-appropriate indulging movement patterns (flow adjustments, low intensity and graduality) on the left side of the tension-flow attribute diagram (Figure 1, diagram 2). The stability needed to maintain these body attitudes requires phase-appropriate aggressive movement patterns (even flow, high intensity and abruptness) on the right side of the tension-flow attribute diagram. A lack of aggressive qualities may delay the child's ability to maintain the new body attitude. Three developmental milestones — self-turning, standing and walking — will illustrate potential clinical problems resulting from developmental delays, which can be identified in skewed diagrams throughout the KMP.

Self-Turning

To accomplish self-turning, flow adjustment must be available to the infant. Flow adjustment involves changing the tension level — it is used in adjusting our position to get more comfortable. It indicates pliability and the facility to adjust to new situations. Persons lacking in flow adjustment may react to a new task or situation by freezing in even flow indicating anxiety.

To complete a turn from prone to supine, infants usually follow this sequence:

1. The head turns to one side (the legs can also
      begin a turn).
2. The arm follows, widening toward the same side.
3. The torso begins to twist.
4. The legs complete the action.

Children first learn to turn onto their side, and to remain there by maintaining an even tension level. Their first complete turns may accidentally result from releasing this even tension. Then they learn to turn at will, using flow adjustment from joint to joint, so that their arm does not get stuck beneath them while turning.

Learning to turn may be delayed for many reasons. The child's genetic personality may be lacking in flow adjustment. The primary caretaker may have used minimal flow adjustment while handling the infant, or may have interfered with the child's natural use of this pattern. For instance, if the caretaker turns the infant over whenever it attempts to turn, the infant will cry when it wishes to turn, instead of trying to turn on its own. Such a child may show an excess of even flow and a lack of flow adjustment, and may become demanding and dependent on its caretaker. Children also practice flow adjustment in feeding, by manipulating the spoon to bring pieces of food to the mouth. Caretakers who do not allow children to feed themselves may inhibit these responses.

A child or adult with this developmental delay will lack

flexibility, have difficulty adjusting to external changes, and feel insecure in unfamiliar situations. The goal of the dance/movement therapist will be to help transform this over-stability into the capacity for change and discovery. At first, the patient will be rigid, immobile, and unapproachable; extra time will be needed to gain trust and establish a safe, stable environment.

These patients often respond well to a form of movement empathy called attunement, which involves kinesthetic identification with their muscle tension. For example, the therapist could use palm-to-palm contact to match a patient's even tension flow. Lower and higher tension changes could be gradually introduced, and then slight twists or flow adjustments may be modelled.

The therapist might suggest movements or images involving twisting, flexibility, indirectness, exploration or scattering. Infants can be engaged in games which require flow adjustment, such as Peek-a-Boo, following a favorite toy with their eyes or hand, or imitating funny twisting faces. Children often respond to the idea of moving like animals, such as snakes or fish. Flexible props, such as scarves or ribbon sticks, can also be used. There is much room for creativity on the part of the therapist in eliciting flow adjustment, flexibility and indirectness.

Standing

To stand, children use the aggressive qualities of high intensity and even flow (diagram 2) to pull themselves up while holding onto a stable object (such as a table or crib). Children who lack phase-appropriate high intensity and straining (diagram 3) will not have enough strength (diagram 4) to hold up their full weight. Such children may find walking forward more pleasant than standing, and will lack the feeling of pride in seeing the world from a vertical perspective.

While children first use their arms to pull themselves up, later they squat (shortening – diagram 5) with feet planted firmly, then raise themselves up (lengthening – diagram 6) to a vertical position, with higher intensity in the pelvis. Then their bodies rise up in one piece, with the upper torso and pelvis firmly connected. They cannot wobble in the middle while maintaining stability with high intensity. When they achieve a full command of standing, they use lower intensity in maintaining a standing position.

As with self-turning, the primary caretaker can unknowingly inhibit the child's ability to stand. If a child accidentally breaks something while attempting to stand, and the caretaker responds with anger, the child may associate this anger with standing, and begin to fear independent action. Such a child may cling and look for approval before going anywhere. Disruption can also occur if the caretaker forcefully pulls the child up by the arms to "help" them stand. This may be experienced as a disempowering interference in the child's self-control, reducing their pride in being able to stand unaided.

When children learn to link high intensity with shortening (pushing into standing), and low intensity with lengthening (standing easily without straining), their physical excitability is balanced by their ability to lower and heighten their body without loss of control. A child who does not use this linkage may become stuck in a standing position, in rigid bound flow. Caretakers who try to help by using force will conflict with the child's desire to develop autonomy, leading to temper tantrums. The lack of affinity between high intensity and lengthening may be seen in the child's anger, as in the child who arches stiffly away from the caretaker's embrace.

An enraged child can often be contained by the therapist or caretaker who uses affined, or related but not the same exact movements of the child. Children can get a sense of security and support by being held with strength and even flow, helping them to control their overwhelming feelings. With an adult client prone to rage reactions, the therapist can use relaxation techniques (while they are calm) to teach self-soothing. The client can experience the transition between high and low tension by squeezing and releasing a therapy ball.

Clients who lack the aggressive elements needed for stable standing can learn to develop strength and high intensity through weight-based images. This could include movements in the vertical plane, such as rocking from side to side, or stooping and standing.

Walking

To walk, children must shift from vertical stability to moving sideways and then to walking forward. This sagittal (forward-backward) movement requires new patterns: graduality (diagram 2) and bulging (diagrams 4 & 5), hesitation (diagram 3) and forward movement (diagram 8), deceleration (diagram 4) and advancing (diagram 9). Toddlers are learning to use aggressive qualities of abruptness (diagram 2), suddenness (diagram 3), and acceleration (diagram 4) within the structuring patterns of hollowing (diagram 4 & 5), moving backwards (diagram 8) and retreating (diagram 9). A child who does not use these patterns of time mastery will have difficulty walking.

Delay in walking can be caused by a caretaker who unwittingly pulls the child's arm up when walking side-by-side. The child cannot properly maintain an alignment in the sagittal plane, because their body is suspended in the air. Children also cannot walk in balance with an adult if their pacing is incompatible. A child who falls while walking and is abruptly pulled up by an adult is unable to break the fall by hollowing, and may learn to lag behind.

Adults who as children experienced a walking delay have difficulty with initiation, termination and sequencing of events. The dance/movement therapist may encourage movement themes such as initiating and terminating contact with group members, starting and stopping, rushing and delaying, and sequencing tasks (such as making and going through an obstacle course). The goals might be learning to time needs, to sequence events, and to balance impulsiveness with patience.

Therapeutic Significance of Developmental Transitions

Developmental transitions such as these are especially vulnerable times for a child. An influx of aggression accompanies them, to enable the child to master the new developmental task. This aggression is normal but may produce behaviors which are difficult to live with, such as biting in the teething phase, throwing in the anal phase or ramming into things in the outer genital phase. An over-reactive response to this aggressive behavior may encourage the child to continue it as a defense. Caretakers can cope by providing acceptable outlets to express aggression. For example, give a biting toy to a teething child, and use the toy to redirect them when they bite another child.

When a trauma occurs in childhood, normal development is disrupted and the adult patient typically retains the issues, defenses and movement patterns characteristic of that stage into adulthood. In the teething phase, biting may be retained as a defense; biting rhythms and oral aggressive patterns (diagram 1) may dominate. Or, biting may be inhibited, and an eating disorder may develop. Such disturbances would be indicated in the KMP by a skewed ratio of teething phase movement patterns.

The therapist can identify the developmental phase associated with the client's aggression, and help them express it in an appropriate, safe environment. In one group dance/movement therapy session for acute psychiatric patients, a schizophrenic woman paced continually, as she did on the unit. The therapist incorporated her pacing into a group movement interaction, using her abrupt rhythm of moving and stopping suddenly, which normally appears in two and a half year-old toddlers in the urethral-sadistic phase of development. The patient was asked to lead a portion of the group session which involved moving to music and stopping when the music was turned off. The patient was invited to be the one to control when the music was playing and when it was stopped. She became extremely animated during this segment of the session, which was in keeping with her preferred movement quality of urethral sadistic rhythms. In this way, she was able to channel her pacing into a movement sequence. She responded very favorably to this suggestion because it used the stop-start aggressive rhythm appropriate to her developmental level.

In general, the therapeutic procedure is to first establish rapport with the patient, and then to facilitate the development of the patient's missing movement patterns. The dance/movement therapist who is trained in the KMP and movement development uses it as an outline to understand the sequence of normal movement patterns in evaluation and treatment planning.

Therapeutic Intervention in the Mother-Child Relationship

In parent-child therapy and in the therapeutic nursery, clinical interventions are often directed at improving the mutual adaptation of mother and child by fostering mutuality, reciprocity and attunement. According to Winnicott (1965), the therapist's place is in the "potential space" between the baby and the mother. The therapeutic nursery is a playground of this potential space, an intermediate area in which the therapeutic staff can facilitate healthy parent-child relationships. Frame-by-frame microanalysis of early parent-child interaction (Beebe & Stern, 1977; Stern, 1971; Brazelton, Koslowski & Main, 1974) has discovered a great deal about early affective and social experience. It has shown the importance for the infant of control over the flow of information and stimulation. Brazelton, Tronick, Adamson et. al., refer to the chaotic non-synchrony (1975, p. 148) in a disturbed mother-child interaction, which manifests as pathology, such as failure to thrive.

The rhythm and movement attunement between parent and child is examined, to determine if the mutually regulated feedback system has been distorted, possibly indicating a serious emotional disturbance. Intervention begins at the point where the connection has been distorted. Children, such as rejecting infants, can bring aberrant behavior into the system (Thoman, 1975). The therapist will try to use (and maximize) the power of the parent-child dyad, to create corrective experiences. The KMP provides an observational language for schematizing their movement patterns, and is an invaluable tool in diagnosis and treatment planning.

Empathy and Trust

While empathy is attunement to another's needs and feelings, as expressed in tension-flow, trust is the adjustment of one's responses to create coordination and predictability, as expressed in shape-flow (Kestenberg & Buelte 1977a, b). A safe holding environment is necessary before either empathy or trust can be created and maintained, whether in the therapeutic alliance or in a mother-child relationship. The primary therapist, as a third element in this dysfunctional relationship, tries to facilitate the development of empathy and trust. This requires being translator, mediator and protector for both sides, and creating a holding environment (sometimes literally) for the parent, so that they, in turn, can provide it for the child. As Kestenberg and Buelte (1977a) have observed, holding another without being held oneself is not conducive to healthy development.

Trust and mistrust become object-directed when shape-flow matures into directional shaping (Kestenberg & Buelte, 1977a). The child's spatial configurations are modelled on the mother's shaping in planes in her embrace and support of the child. Trustful and distrustful feelings develop in shape-flow. For example, a bipolar shape-flow skewed toward narrowing, shortening and hollowing, with little growing, indicates poor narcissistic development, and small, uneasy or empty feelings about self.

Continued healthy development will involve conflict as well as attunement between parent and child, depending on the child's stage of maturity (cf. Kestenberg, 1965, 1975). Complete attunement and tension-flow synchronicity become maladaptive once the symbiotic phase has passed. It is important to remember that clashing and individuated patterns are necessary for the construction of healthy ego boundaries. When these conflicts are not able to develop, pathology may result. For instance, some schizophrenic patients show an uncanny empathy, an ability to identify the needs and feelings of others (including the therapist). Their capacity for affective merger is over-developed and inappropriately directed; their tension-flow attunement is extreme, one-sided and generally unsustainable. Our current impression (requiring further study) is that a subgroup of patients are inclined to show heightened attunement in tension-flow and extremely limited adjustment in shape-flow (i.e., "I feel what you feel; I don't trust you"). Another subgroup, fearing merger, cannot tolerate attunement experiences.

To see how such skews may occur, take the example of a mother holding her baby in bound flow and high anxiety. Her anxiety flows only one way, toward her child, and limits her ability to receive emotional feedback. Her baby's ability to attune with her is therefore restricted; she can only feel the child's emotion when it is the same as hers. Lacking true empathy, the baby experiences a one-sided symbiosis, encouraging it to develop a false sense of self (Winnicott, 1965). This interactive perspective may be applied to patients across the diagnostic spectrum. In severe disturbances, the patient's one-sided empathy also lacks feelings of trust and comfort. A sense of sameness develops without a sense of relatedness, because the other person is not experienced as reciprocally adjusting. This, in turn, requires defenses against these frightening feelings.

Empathy and trust can also be diagnostically useful. In one case, empathic attunement revealed an inaccurate diagnosis, which otherwise might not have been discovered. The patient was an elderly woman with a profound loss of cognitive and memory functioning, diagnosed with dementia by her psychiatrist, psychologist and neurologist. From a movement perspective, she exhibited a lot of neutral flow (wooden or limp movement, shapelessness and lack of body boundaries), which is associated with depression, illness and fatigue. Movement therapy using hand-to-hand tension-flow attunement was begun as a prelude to experimental treatment with cognitive stimulation. However, in the course of the attunement therapy, her ability to establish a relationship re-emerged, she became more verbal, and her memory functioning improved significantly. The experimental techniques were never implemented, and eventually psychotherapy was used effectively. Her diagnosis was retroactively revised to severe depression manifesting as pseudodementia.

However, attunement alone is no more sufficient for therapy than it is for ego-development. The therapist wishes to communicate not only empathy and understanding, but also support, structure and confidence. An enraged client in high-intensity even flow who hears a response in low-intensity flow adjustment such as "don't worry, it's all right," is unlikely to feel understood. On the other hand, a therapist who becomes equally enraged and anxious destroys the therapeutic holding environment. The KMP provides a framework for understanding the complexity of this situation: mirroring, contrasting and affined patterns must all be appropriately combined to provide an effective therapeutic response.

Clashing patterns during early feeding experiences are particularly important, as this is when children learn to regulate their intake; the clashes may lead to eating disorders later (cf. Charone, 1982). Consider this scenario: a 13-month old boy is sitting face-to-face with his mother, who is feeding him with a spoon. His tension-flow expresses graduality, low intensity flow-adjustment and indirectness, as his attention wanders around the room. His mother becomes frustrated by her perceived failure at feeding. She narrows her brow and shoulders, raising her level of intensity and abruptness. In aggressive bound flow, containing her impulses, she blocks out everything except channeling the spoon toward his mouth. This clashing pattern is continually repeated, especially during feeding. Sometimes it precipitates a temper tantrum, but just as often they appear to meet in a kind of neutral zone, without making true contact, and the task is completed with a striking lack of relatedness. The solution of meeting in a neutral zone is not uncommon; it is often seen when the mother is severely depressed. The child seems to find that this neutrality is the only place to connect, even minimally, with the mother.

Autism and the KMP

The KMP has great potential for use in early at-risk assessment, treatment planning, and research with autistic children. This section is intended to stimulate the development of further applications of the KMP to autism. Future research with the KMP can produce more definitive descriptions of autistic children (and other diagnostic groups). Especially needed are correlational studies using other measures of descriptive appraisal (such as BRIAAC — Ruttenberg, Kalish, Wenar et al, 1974). It is possible that research with populations characterized by repetitive, stereotypic movement patterns may require amended profiling procedures to account for their skewed frequency distributions (perhaps scoring stereotypic and nonstereotypic behavior separately as two distinct profiles).

Behavioral Description

Children with pervasive developmental disorders, such as early onset infantile autism, generally show atypical, repetitive movement patterns along with gross impairment in interpersonal responsiveness and communication skills. Common autistic movements include grimacing, rocking, arm-flapping, and jumping up and down. They are exacerbated by any stimulation, such as a spinning toy (cf. Wing, 1975). Other movements found in autistic children include rocking from back foot to front foot while bending at the waist, walking on tip-toe, body spinning, odd postures, etc. In one autistic case, Kestenberg noted "his very peculiar body schema... [His legs showed fluidity and] were very much his own [while the upper part of his body was in] fixed control [and was] rejected as nonexistent and later as not belonging to him" (1954, pp. 37-38).

Neutral Flow

The typically limp, Raggedy Ann-like body attitude of autistic children is due to their excessive neutrality of tension-flow and shape-flow, a lack of both elasticity and plasticity. This manifests as floppiness, sometimes alternating with rigidity, blankness, a lack of kinesthetic animation, and inertia. Although they may episodically break out of neutral flow, they always return to it. In adults, excessive neutral flow can be found in severe depression, in extreme catatonia, in fatigue and in altered states of consciousness. Neutral shape-flow involves a loss of body boundaries; the autistic child's body appears to dissolve. On the other hand, autistic children often create and maintain intense bound tension on the periphery (i.e., finger twisting). Perhaps this creates primitive body boundaries where otherwise there are none.

It is normal to use some level of neutral tension-flow, particularly in relating to inanimate objects. However, autistic children appear to use neutral tension-flow to become inanimate themselves, like wheels or other spinning objects. This poses a problem for the therapist who wishes to enter this discomforting, non-feeling world and attune with the child. According to Kestenberg, it is necessary to enter into a neutral zone to establish contact (Kestenberg & Buelte, 1977a, b). The child regulates the contact in the neutral zone, and then is able to expand contact into give-and-take games. Since autistic children show little or no imitation, the therapist will imitate them (kinesthetic contact is preferable to visual contact). In this attunement, both child and therapist will use the most basic tension-flow attributes before moving up the developmental line.

Localization of Tension

Localized tension-flow is a developmental prototype of gesture which initiates and maintains flow changes in functionally related body zones, as in sucking (Kestenberg & Sossin, 1979). Its counterpart is centralized flow, which spreads flow changes through contiguous regions of the body. In autistic children, centralized flow is inhibited; their flow appears to be highly localized, except in ritualized discharges, where high-intensity bound flow and abruptness occur throughout the body. Localized flow appears to be involved in their segmented and isolated repetitive patterns, their lack of movement continuity, and their use of apparently clashing patterns or unrelated patterns in different parts of the body.

Partial Stabilization of Tension

Stabilization of tension decreases the frequency of flow changes. Complete stabilization would mean immobility throughout the body, so normal development leads to functionally adaptive partial stabilization. This reduces flow changes to limit interference with localized motor discharges and gestures (like fixing in movement therapy, which stabilizes one body part to promote mobility elsewhere). Excessive stabilization can be seen in cases where rigidity interferes with normal mobility. Excessive mobilization can be seen in Attention Deficit Disorder with hyperactivity. Localization and partial stabilization are distinct but related processes. In some disabilities, an intense and exaggerated overuse of partial stabilization is developed as a compensation for the loss of the localization function.

Partial stabilization seems largely undeveloped in autistic

children, despite their high level of localization. Their mobility appears detached; they use neutral flow in place of partial stabilization. A rush of sudden aggressive high-intensity and affined shrinking (such as bipolar hollowing and shortening) may sweep through their entire body, without any recognizable environmental stimulus. Such episodes vividly illustrate their lack of functional regulation through partial stabilization.

Other Autistic Features

The characteristic grimaces and flapping patterns of autistic children have several other distinctive features, as defined by the KMP. Shape-flow will be used as an example. One autistic child freqently used an oblique facial gesture with unipolar shortening, hollowing and widening of the mouth, accentuated by medial narrowing, in high intensity of tension. The discomfort of shrinking clashing with widening in aggressive high intensity signalled to others an aversion to interpersonal contact, and served to break off communication.

This characteristic repulsion of interpersonal stimuli in autistic children is accompanied by a preference for shrinking patterns of shape-flow. Closed, shrinking bipolar patterns also provide the structure for inwardly-directed aggression, such as bruxism (teeth grinding), self-biting and self-hitting. Exhalation is more pronounced than inhalation in the autistic child's breathing rhythm (Blau & Siegel, 1978) reflecting greater shrinking than growing patterns. Not surprisingly, they usually do not show any shaping in planes, reflecting their lack of multi-dimensional object relations. Only after the development of object constancy will the autistic child begin to show shaping in planes.

Therapeutic Implications

The fundamental questions about the nature of autism have split the field into separate camps; an integrated conceptualization of its etiology is still in the future, and may involve several factors. Biomedical research on the treatment of autism has been progressing slowly since the late 1960's (Cohen & Shaywitz, 1982; Campbell, Cohen & Anderson, 1981). Observation and case studies have increased our understanding of the psychodynamic and psychogenic factors in autism (Tustin, 1981). This has led to an appreciation of the autistic state as a powerful shield aginst feelings of separation, and has produced psychotherapeutic techniques to help children develop filtering mechanisms for perceptual, kinesthetic and interpersonal experience.

In autism, the child's bond with the primary caretaker does not evolve normally. Treatment approaches can be based on developmental movement patterns (Adler, 1968; Kalish, 1968), such as the KMP. A treatment strategy incorporating the KMP was used for a three-year old autistic boy at a therapeutic nursery. It aimed to facilitate interaction between mother and child, in the nursery and at home. This involved both shape-flow patterns affined with the child's tension-flow, and deliberate clashing of shape-flow and tension-flow, to direct aggression outwards. Empathy was facilitated through tension-flow attunement (pushing-pulling and giving-taking games), signing and parental psychotherapy. The boy had less neutral flow and clearer body boundaries than his mother, with spurts of initiation. The mother felt discomfort in neutral flow; this was discussed in therapy, enhancing her empathetic ability. Her growing responsiveness to flow changes led to more attunement in touching and holding her child. The boy then showed more imitation, less localization and less isolation of flow. Improved attunement also led to increased and prolonged eye contact. Mutual breathing between mother and child was also used: rhythmic growing into and separating from each other in all body planes (shape-flow). At first the boy's responses were unpredictable and unreliable, improving as their attunement increased. The normal process of shape-flow adjustment leading to mirroring and identification (Kestenberg & Buelte, 1977a), was seen in the improved relational patterns resulting from shape-flow harmony.

Directions for Future KMP Research

This paper has focused on application of the KMP in dance/movement therapy involving developmental transitions. It has described the KMP's approach to psychological appraisal, and its application in clinical observation and treatment planning. The KMP provides an organic, but sophisticated, framework for the notation, classification, and psychodynamic interpretation of movement patterns. Its systematic observational schema and broad scope of application in assessment, diagnosis and treatment make it an ideal research tool. Knowledge of the KMP and its growing body of research gives the clinician a deeper appreciation and understanding of preverbal and nonverbal behavior.

Further research will enable the KMP to evolve as a clinical tool; so far, its developmental model has been primarily based on hundreds of case studies, including longitudinal studies, of children, adolescents and adults (Kestenberg, 1965a & b, 1967; Kestenberg & Sossin, 1979). The KMP's interpretive framework and clinical utility will develop as it is applied to a broad spectrum of research topics. For instance, future research may be pursued either from a movement perspective or in conjunction with psychoanalytic metapsychology.

Future studies can produce norms for healthy and pathological populations across culture, age and sex, from which a statistical outline of diagnostic indicators can be drawn. Longitudinal research with the KMP can advance psychodynamic theory by tracing specific developmental issues (such as aggression, narcissism, superego development or personality) from early infancy. Detailed studies of specific diagnostic populations are needed to establish the range of individual variation within groups. Other subjects for study could include premature infants, individuals with physical illnesses, role-dependent or context-dependent behavior. Research using the KMP may improve our understanding of the borderline personality. It could compare the borderline personality's pre-genital aggression and lack of object synthesis (Kernberg, 1975), with the rages of the auto-aggressive child (Mahler, 1968). More research can also increase our understanding of risk factors, prevention and early intervention approaches with vulnerable infants and children (Kestenberg & Buelte, 1983).

Methodological research can examine the reliability of the current notation (Sossin, 1987), and develop amended profiling procedures as needed for specific applications. Computer programs can facilitate scoring and correlation of profiles. The validity of the current interpretive schema can be examined, and specific distributions can be related to clinically-relevant variables such as IQ, depression, neurological impairment, defense mechanisms, and systemic conflicts.

Simplified Graphic Representation of the KMP

This profile (Figure 1) of a 13-month old boy illustrates some of the risk features for a young child. His tension-flow rhythms show a disproportionate ratio of sadistic to libidinal tension-flow rhythms (the right side vs. the left side) and notable amounts of urethral sadistic (run-stop-go) rhythms, both pure (solid lines) and mixed (broken lines). Studies indicate that the latter feature may be linked with neurological disturbances when it is not phase-appropriate, as in this anal-phase child.

Another diagnostic feature is the disharmony (clashes and imbalances) between the left side and the right side of the KMP. For example, comparison of precursors of effort with shaping in directions shows three obvious clashes: channeling with sideways movement, vehemence with upward movement, and suddenness with forward movement. These clashes indicate that his defenses against drives (precursors of effort) do not fit well with his defenses against objects (shaping in directions). Simply put, his responses to internal demands (bodily needs) and external demands (environmental stimuli) are incongruous.

An example of imbalance can be seen by comparing the amount of even flow in tension-flow attributes, with the amount of narrowing in bipolar shape-flow. This indicates that there is too much structure (shape-flow) for the amount of dynamic impact (tension-flow attributes) available.

Another indication of possible maladaptation is shown by the extremely low load factors for tension-flow attributes, effort, and shaping in planes (33% is the minimum). His low load factors show a significant lack of complexity in affective expression, adaptation to reality and approach to relationships, respectively. He rarely uses more than one element of motion in these areas.

These indicators, among others, show his vulnerability at this stage of development. Further profiles will need to be done to assess his subsequent developmental progress, and to measure the success of any interventions.

_____

References

Adler, J. (1968). The study of an autistic child (film and presentation). Proceedings of the American Dance Therapy Association, Third Annual Conference (pp. 43-48). Madison, WI: American Dance Therapy Association.

Bartenieff, I., & Lewis, D. (1980). Body movement: Coping with the environment. New York: Gordon and Breach.

Beebe, B., & Stern, D. (1977). Engagement-disengagement and early object experiences. In N. Freedmand & S. Grand (Eds.), Communicative structures and psychic structures. New York: Plenum Press.

Blau, B., & Siegel, E. V. (1978). Breathing together: A preliminary investigation of an involuntary reflex as adaptation. American Journal of Dance Therapy, 2, 35-42.

Brazelton, T. B., Koslowski, B., & Main, M. (1974). The origins of reciprocity. In M. Lewis and L. A. Roseblum (Eds.), The effect of the infant on its caregiver. New York: Wiley-Interscience.

Brazelton, T. B., Tronick, E., Adamson, L., Als, H., & Wise, S. (1975). Early mother-infant reciprocity. In Ciba Foundation Symposium 33: Parent-infant interaction. New York: American Elsevier.

Bridges, Laurel (1989). Measuring the effect of dance/movement therapy on the body image of institutionalized elderly using the Kestenberg Movement Profile and projective drawings. Unpublished master's thesis, Antioch New England Graduate School, Keene, NH.

Campbell, M., Cohen, I. L., & Anderson, L.T. (1981). Pharmacotherapy for autistic children: A summary of research. Canadian Journal of Psychiatry, 26, 265-273.

Charone, J. K. (1982). Eating disorders: Their genesis in the mother-infant relationship. International Journal of Eating Disorders, 1, 15-42.

Cohen, D. J., & Shaywitz, B. A. (1982). Preface to special issue on neurobiological research in autism. Journal of Autism and Developmental Disorders, 12, 103-108.

Dosamantes, E. (1990). Movement and psychodynamic pattern changes in long-term dance/movement therapy groups. American Journal of Dance Therapy, 12, 27-44.

Freud, A. (1965). Normality and pathology in childhood: Assessments of development. In The writings of Anna Freud (Vol. 6). New York: International Universities Press.

Kalish, B. (1968). Body movement therapy for autistic children. Proceedings of the American Dance Therapy Association, Third Annual Conference (pp. 49-59). Madison, WI: American Dance Therapy Association.

Kernberg, O. (1975). Borderline conditions and pathological narcissism. New York: Jason Aronson.

Kestenberg, J. S. (1954). The history of an "autistic child": Clinical data and interpretation. Journal of Child Psychiatry, 2, 5-52.

Kestenberg, J. S. (1965a). The role of movement patterns in development: 1. Rhythms of movement. Psychoanalytic Quarterly, 34, 1-36.

Kestenberg, J. S. (1965b). The role of movement patterns in development: 2. Flow of tension and effort. Psychoanalytic Quarterly, 34, 517-563.

Kestenberg, J. S. (1966). Rhythm and organization in obsessive-compulsive development. International Journal of Psychoanalysis, 47, 151-159.

Kestenberg, J. S. (1967). The role of movement patterns in development: 3. The control of shape. Psychoanalytic Quarterly, 36, 356-409.

Kestenberg, J. S. (1971). From organ-object imagery to self- and-object representations. In J. B. McDevitt (Ed.), Separation-individuation: Papers in honor of Margaret Mahler. New York: International Universities Press.

Kestenberg, J. S. (1975). Children and parents. New York: Jason Aronson.

Kestenberg, J. S. (1976). Regression and reintegration in pregnancy. Journal of the American Psychoanalytic Association, 24, 213-250.

Kestenberg, J. S. (1980a). Ego-organization in obsessive- compulsive development: A study of the Rat-Man, based on interpretation of movement patterns. In M. Kanzer & J. Glenn (Eds.), Freud and his patients. New York: Jason

Aronson.

Kestenberg, J. S. (1980b). The inner-genital phase — prephallic and preoedipal. In D. Mendel (Ed.), Early feminine development: Contemporary psychoanalytic views. New York: Spectrum Publications.

Kestenberg, J. S. (1985). The flow of empathy and trust between mother and child. In E. J. Anthony and G. H. Pollack (Eds.), Parental influences: In health and disease. pp. 137-163. Boston: Little Brown.

Kestenberg, J. S., & Buelte, A. (1977a). Prevention, infant therapy and the treatment of adults: 1. Toward understanding mutuality. International Journal of Psychoanalytic Psychotherapy, 6, 339-366.

Kestenberg, J. S., & Buelte, A. (1977b). Prevention, infant therapy and the treatment of adults: 2. Mutual holding and holding-oneself-up. International Journal of Psychoanalytic Psychotherapy, 6, 369-396.

Kestenberg, J. S., & Buelte, A. (1983). Prevention, infant therapy and the treatment of adults: 3. Periods of vulnerability in transitions from stability to mobility and vice versa. In J. Call, E. Galenson, and R. Tyson (Eds.), Frontiers of Infant Psychiatry. New York: Basic Books.

Kestenberg, J. S., & Marcus, H. (1979). Hypothetical monosex and bisexuality. In M. C. Nelson & J. Ikenberry (Eds.), Psychosexual imperatives. New York: Human Sciences Press.

Kestenberg, J. S., Marcus, H., Robbins, E., Berlowe, J., & Buelte, A. (1971). Development of the young child as expressed through bodily movement. Journal of the American Psychoanalytic Association, 19, 746-764.

Kestenberg, J. S., Marcus, H., Sossin, K. M., & Stevenson, R. (1982). The development of paternal attitudes. In S. Cath, A. Gurwitt & J. Ross (Eds.), Fathers: Observations and reflections. Boston: Little-Brown.

Kestenberg, J. S., & Sossin, K. M. (1979). The role of movement patterns in development (Vol. 2). New York: Dance Notation Bureau Press.

Kestenberg, J. S., & Weinstein, J. (1978). Transitional objects and body image formation. In S. A. Grolnick, L. Barkin & W. Muensterberger (Eds.), Between reality and fantasy:

Transitional objects and phenomena. New York: Jason Aronson.

Laban, R., & Lawrence, F. C. (1947). Effort. London: MacDonald & Evans.

Laban, R. (1960) The mastery of movement (2nd ed.). London: MacDonald & Evans.

Lamb, W. (1965). Posture and gesture. London: Gerald Duckworth.

Lamb, W. & Watson, E. (1987). Body code: The meaning in movement (2nd ed.). Princeton, NJ: Princeton Book Company, Publishers.

Lemon, Janet (1990). The use of dance movement therapy in professional sport. Unpublished master's thesis, Antioch New England Graduate School, Keene, NH.

Lewis, P., (Ed.), (1984). Theoretical approaches in dance-movement therapy, Vol.II. (2nd ed.). Dubuque, IA: W.C. Brown-Kendall/Hunt Publishing Co.

Lewis, P., (Ed.), (1986). Theoretical approaches in dance-movement therapy, Vol.I. Dubuque, IA: W.C. Brown-Kendall/Hunt Publishing Co.

Lewis, P. (1990) The Kestenberg Movement Profile in the psychotherapeutic process with borderline disorders. In P. Lewis & S. Loman (Eds.), The Kestenberg Movement Profile, its past, present applications, and future directions. Keene, NH: Antioch New England Graduate School.

Loman, S. (1991). Refining movement interventions in dance/movement therapy: a model of nonverbal interaction utilising the Kestenberg Movement Profile (KMP) system of movement analysis. In Shadow & light: Moving toward wholeness. Columbia, MD: American Dance Therapy Association.

Mahler, M. S. (1968). On human symbiosis and the vicissitudes of individuation. New York: International Universities Press.

Ramsden, P. (1973). Top team planning. New York: Halsted/Wiley.

Ruttenberg, B., Kalish, B., Wenar, C., & Wolf, E. (1974). A description of the Behavior Rating Instrument for Autistic and other Atypical Children (BRIAAC). Therapeutic process: Movement as integration: Proceedings of the Ninth Annual

Conference (pp. 139-142). New York: American Dance Therapy Association.

Sandel, S. L. (1982). The process of individuation in dance-movement therapy with schizophrenic patients. The Arts in Psychotherapy, 9, 11-18.

Siegel, E. V. (1974). Psychoanalytic thought and methodology in dance movement therapy. Focus on Dance, 7, 27-37.

Siegel, E. V. (1984). Dance movement therapy: mirror of our selves and the psychoanalytic approach. New York: Human Sciences Press.

Sossin, K. M. (1987). Reliability of the Kestenberg Movement Profile. Movement Studies: Observer Agreement, vol 2, 23-28. New York: Laban/Bartenieff Institute of Movement Studies.

Stern, D. N. (1971). A micro-analysis of mother-infant interaction: Behavior regulating social contact between a mother and her three and a half month-old twins. Journal of the American Academy of Child Psychiatry, 10, 501-517.

Thoman, E. (1975). How a rejecting baby affects mother-infant synchrony. In Ciba Foundation Symposium 33: Parent-infant interaction. New York: American Elsevier.

Tustin, F. (1981). Autistic states in children. London: Routledge & Kegan Paul.

Wing, L. (1975). Diagnosis, clinical description and prognosis. In L. Wing (Ed.), Early childhood autism (2nd ed.). Oxford, England: Pergamon Press.

Winnicott, D. W. (1965). The maturational processes and the facilitating environment. New York: Internation Univeristies Press.

The Use of Expressive Arts in Prevention: Facilitating the Construction of Objects

Judith S. Kestenberg, M.D.

The choreographer and dancer Rudolf Laban, known for his invention of Labanotation and effort notation, was first a painter. When he turned to dance, he became interested in the live pictures on stage. He distinguished between stable and mobile patterns of movement, and he linked visual art and music to movement:

> Movement is the first and most basic language that man uses to express his inner wishes and experiences. One must always remember that *all tones*, as in speaking, singing and screaming, *stem from bodily actions, that is, movement.* Whether I hit the table so that it resonates or make the air tremble with my scream, it is always the same, namely movement made audible (1935, p. 112; *italics added,* author's translation).

Laban described himself as a man with a sense of vision and a sense of form. Freud was a master of both. Using the teachings of Laban and Freud, the Sands Point Movement Study Group (Robbins, Marcus, Berlowe, Buelte and myself) constructed a movement profile from which one can make a psychological assessment of the mover, modelled after that introduced by Anna Freud (1965). Using this profile, we can detect patterns in everyday movements of infants and their parents, and can also find these patterns in pictorial and three-dimensional art products as well as in music, "the audible movement."

In this paper, I shall give a brief overview of movement patterns which can be observed in visual art, dance and music. Concentrating primarily on visual art, I will illustrate this in brief vignettes of three Renaissance masterpieces, all of which have also been interpreted by Freud. I will then introduce the principles of preventing emotional disorders via expressive art, with particular emphasis on the construction and reconstruction of object- and self-images. In the last part, I will try to demonstrate through babies' and toddlers' drawings how bodily feelings are expressed at different phases in the formation of a body scheme (Schilder, 1935/1950).

The Flow of Tension

Elasticity is ubiquitous within all living tissue, and is manifested in the flow of tension (tension-flow) in movement and at rest. The fetus and the newborn alternate between rigidity and freedom, in the vital rhythm of **bound** and **free flow.** Through bound flow, we inhibit movement, and this inhibition becomes the prototype of most defensive actions. Through free flow, we mobilize ourselves and indulge in the freedom of our actions. The various combinations of bound and free flow give vent to feelings ranging from anxiety to carefreeness. Freely flowing movement expresses ease of mind and can also be seen in the freely flowing lines of a drawing, or heard in freely flowing sequences of music and dance. Normally, free and bound flow alternate in a repetitive fashion, thus creating the substrate for rhythms. Every quality can be repeated in a rhythmic fashion, but no matter what these qualities are, whether swinging movements, lines and loops in a drawing, or tones and beats in music, they all ride on waves of tension-flow which have been made subservient to their special aims. When we feel poised, unruffled or steady, we move in **even flow** of tension; when we make a change or adjust to something new, feeling squirmy or playful, we use an **adjustment of tension** level. When our feelings are intense, we have a **high intensity** of tension, and when we calm ourselves, this recedes to a **low intensity** of tension. When we act impulsively, we are using an **abrupt** change of tension, but when we are patient, we are using a **gradual** change of tension.

Figure 1. Michaelangelo's "Moses"

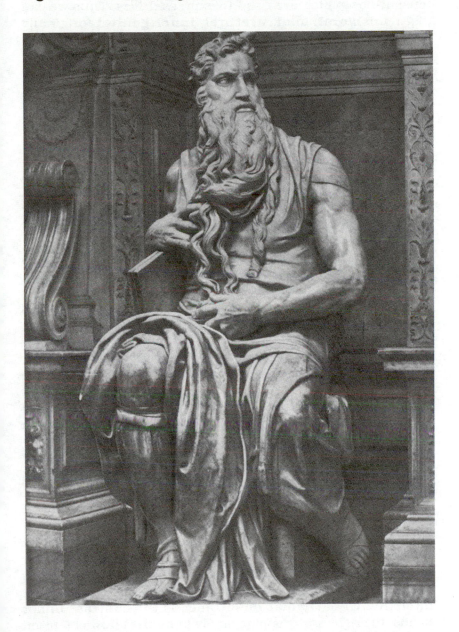

The repetition of certain flow sequences creates rhythms of tension-flow which are used to express drives. Thus we can distinguish **oral**, **anal**, **urethral**, **inner-genital** (originally called feminine) and **outer-genital** (originally called phallic) rhythms of tension-flow.

In Michaelangelo's "Moses" (Figure 1), almost all of the body is in highly bound tension, indicating that he is holding back anger. This contrasts with the lower tension of his fingers, which play with his long beard. There is even higher tension in the nape of his neck, his gaze and his torso, as well as in his right leg, and there is quite a bit of tension-flow adjustment (twisting kind) in the fold of his beard. Here we also see an inner-genital type of gradually ascending low tension rhythms, repeated in the horizontal folds of his clothing. However, the vertical folds are predominant; they have an outer-genital character.

This description of tension-flow fits well with Freud's interpretation of the statue. Freud (1914/1955) concludes that Michaelangelo's Moses was holding onto the God-given tablets to prevent himself from dropping them in anger. In Freud's view, when Moses discovered the worship of the golden calf, he grabbed his beard forcefully, turning his aggression inward. At this moment, the tablets began to slip from his grip. Rather than throwing and breaking them, as described in the Bible, he re-established his grip on the tablets, and in this process had to let go of his beard, so that only the right forefinger remained entangled (although his middle finger also seems to be deep in the beard). Freud thought that Michaelangelo was rebuilding the image of Moses and of his patron, the pope, making them compassionate rather than ruthless, patient rather than impulsive.

In the face of Mona Lisa (Figure 2), we see flow adjustment at the corners of her mouth and cheeks. This gives her smile a benign, playful character. What makes it so enigmatic is its contrast with the even flow in the rest of her body, particularly her forehead. High intensity in bound flow can be detected in her gaze, but also a graduality that softens the impact of her intensity. Of particular importance is the contrast in her hands, the right one dropping limply in **neutral flow** of tension over the left one that holds the book in bound, even flow. Freud

Figure 2. da Vinci's Mona Lisa

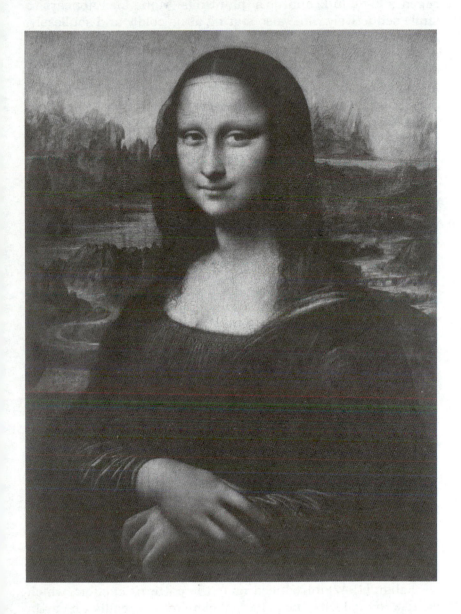

commented that no one had solved the riddle of the smile that repeats itself in Leonardo's paintings. Mona Lisa appears to smile seductively while also staring at us coldly and soullessly. He quotes Muentz, who said that Mona Lisa expresses the very essence of femininity. Why should the clash between staring coldly (bound, even flow) and smiling seductively (adjustment in low intensity of tension) be seen as feminine? To be sure, it does encompass the contradictory nature traditionally ascribed to women, but does this really add up to the concept of femininity?

The impression of archetypal femininity is given by the repetition of the predominant rhythmic inner-genital waves, radiating from inside out and curving her face, her arms and hands, the folds of her clothing, her veil and the rhythmically positioned curls of her hair. In these waves we see low intensity and graduality of tension-flow that conveys femininity, in addition to rhythms in her body, her clothes and the landscape, all of which can be interpreted as feminine.

Freud quotes Herzfeld, who declared that "in the Mona Lisa, Leonardo encountered his own self . . . [her] features had lain all along in mysterious sympathy within Leonardo's mind" (1910/1957, p. 110). This implies that Leonardo was in tune with the tension-flow of his subject, so that he could paint what she felt. Such an attunement is the physical core of empathy between mother and child (Kestenberg & Buelte, 1977). Freud stated that from his youth on, Leonardo was attracted towards "portraying . . . two kinds of objects . . . [and if] the beautiful childrens' heads were reproductions of his own person as it was in his childhood, then the smiling women are nothing other than the repetitions of his mother Catherina" (1910/1957, p. 111), whom Leonardo had to leave when he was three to five years old.

Laban's Efforts of Space, Weight and Time and Langer's Virtual Space and Time

Laban (1947) introduced us to the patterns of effort, which we use to deal with the principal elements of reality on earth: space, by **direct** or **indirect** movements, gravity or weight, by **strong** or **light** movements, and time, by **acceleration** or

deceleration. Through their control over tension-flow, efforts can harness the expression of affects and incorporate them into actions, thereby dealing with reality affectively.

Using even flow as an affective core, Mona Lisa looks at us directly, but her smile, her cheeks and the angles of her eyelids suggest an indirect approach, one that is not as forthright and precise as her direct gaze. There is a lightness about her that makes us want to smile and soar with her, but the boundness of her torso and the fingers of her left hand inhibit this impulse.

Although all the different types of tension-flow can be incorporated in the various patterns of effort, there is an optimal resonance between certain types of affective expression and modes of dealing with reality. The term resonance indicates that one movement instrument resonates with another to form a complex, pleasing entity in which feelings and adaptive behavior are optimally integrated (Kestenberg & Sossin, 1979). Thus, direct movement arises from even tension-flow, and indirectness from tension-flow adjustment. Strength rides on high intensity of tension and lightness on low intensity. Acceleration springs from abruptness and deceleration from graduality. Music, too, can spread through space directly or indirectly, with strength or lightness, with acceleration or deceleration, and these effort elements can merge harmoniously with the corresponding feeling tones emanating from the melody. In visual art, the artist's feelings, expressed through tension-flow, and their adaptation to reality, expressed through effort, leave residues of these motion factors on canvas.

The great strength of Michaelangelo's "Moses" is coordinated with a very high intensity of tension. His wrath is controlled by his strength and determination. The fighting, contending effort of strength is mitigated by the indulging indirectness that can be seen in the way his limbs seem to have moved in space. In contrast, the direct look in his eyes indicates the concentrated attention with which he views the sin of his people. Through maintaining the intensity of his tension-flow, he keeps himself steady, and levels his feelings, while at the same time attending to what is best for all.

Leonardo's "Madonna and Child with St. Anne" (Figure 3),

Figure 3. da Vinci's Madonna and Child with St. Anne

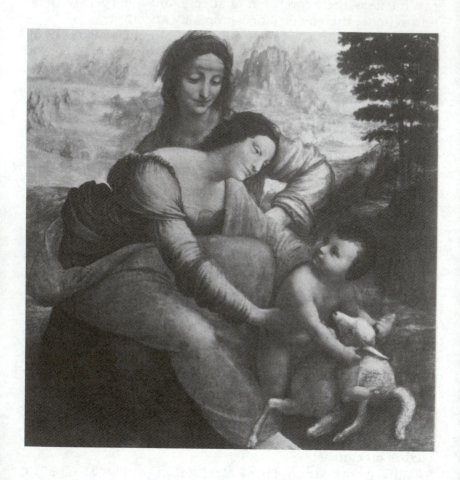

expresses indirectness through the positions of the moving limbs of the Madonna and Child. At the same time, we see a continuous adjustment of tension levels, not only in the graduated smiles of the three figures, but also in the bodies of the Madonna and Child. This contrasts with the immobile, bound arm of St. Anne: despite her loving and gentle facial expression, she keeps her distance, remaining unruffled, poised and scrutinizing. Her arm reveals a direct approach rather than an accomodating one, although her face promises flexibility.

Susan Langer (1953) defined the impression of space in visual art and the impression of time in music as virtual space and virtual time, respectively. From the psychoanalytic perspective, these ideas can be conceptualized as internalized space and internalized time. Incongruously, both Langer (1953) and Laban (1920) identify gesture as the primary symbolic vehicle of dance. **Gesture** is created by movement in a part or parts of the body (Lamb, 1965), which traverses space in trace forms and acts as a signifier or symbol in communication. It is largely determined by culture and represents a category quite different from those of space and time. This basic error is shared by almost all writers who focus on space and time and neglect the element of gravity (one notable exception is Schilder, 1935/1950). Despite this blind spot, both Langer and Laban come close to the true essence of dance: virtual gravity, derived from the experience of weight. Langer refers to the "quite genuine virtual powers" (1953, p. 202) created even in social dance. She also speaks of the "powers of traditional mystic dancing, vaguely distinguishable from erotic forces, the bonds of love and the communing selves, or *the freedom from gravity*" (italics added). Laban said that dance is bound to the earth and consists always of the change from stillness to stir, "between the held equilibrium on a point of support" and the act of breaking away from it (1971, p. 62). He enjoined his students to remember that hopping was our first attempt to dance, that is, to get away from the earth.

Freud has spoken of the inevitable disappointment to our narcissistic omnipotence when we realized that the earth is only one of many planets in the solar system, revolving around the much larger sun; and again, when we realized that we cannot control our unconscious. Perhaps it is a similiar disappointment with our inability to fly that has made it so difficult for art theorists, psychologists and philosophers to come to terms with the force of gravity. Freud linked dreams and wishes about flying with erotic feelings, especially those arising from the phallus. No doubt, there are erotic components to experiences of flying through the air, of being tossed in the air by our parents, or being carried through space by parental arms; but our life-long struggle with the force of gravity, experienced as pull or weight, also has an adaptive component. Being pressed to the parent's body, then getting away from it; swaying upwards and flying away, then returning; being moved rhythmically and feeling one's own weight: all are reproduced in dance. Abstracted from body feelings and body mass and internalized, it becomes virtual gravity.

Although all effort qualities are used in every art form, each of the three art media discussed here focuses on a dominant effort range: space, in visual art; gravity, in dance; and time, in music. We must remember that these are the primary ingredients of our external reality.

Most discussants of art (Arnheim, 1969; Gardner, 1980; Kris, 1952) speak of art as expressing feelings and/or creating reality in one sense or another. However, neither feelings nor reality can be re-created in a vacuum, void of objects. Art allows us to create objects within the context of inner feelings and external reality.

The Flow of Shape

While tension-flow is based on the biological properties of contractility and elasticity, **shape-flow** refers to the properties of living tissue, in the areas of expandability and plasticity. Shape-flow gives form to tension-flow as we **grow** or **shrink** in shape in flowing between free and bound flow (Lamb, 1965). Shapes are framed by space, but they have their own expandable and constrictable boundaries within which we feel **wide**, large and generous or **narrow**, constricted and needy; **lengthened**, big and important or **shortened**, small and insignificant; **bulging** and full or **hollow** and empty. Our breathing, growing in inhalation and shrinking in exhalation, supports not only our quest for survival on a body level, but also underlies our mimetics and those gestures which act as signals for help from others.

If our affective expressions are to be understood, certain rules must be observed. For instance, if you try to smile during exhalation, you will not produce a smile, but rather a grin. Smiling widens your face, while exhalation tends to shrink your body shape. There is a congruence between inhalation and growing and between exhalation and shrinking.

Alterations in shape-flow make feelings meaningful in a number of ways. Interpreters of drawings are aware that tiny figure drawings on a large page betray the drawer's feelings of insignificance. It is not difficult to recognize the role of shape in a dancer's body, but we are much less familiar with interpreting the shape of a singer, especially when we hear the song but do not see the singer. We can, with some training, guess how big or small the singer's vocal chords are, and how their shape changes as the pitch varies. We recognize the location and shape of the spaces in the body which resonate more than others during singing (Shields & Robbins, 1980). We can estimate the amount of air being pressed through the opening of the vocal chords. We can sense whether the singer is projecting, growing toward the audience; or singing inwards, as if shrinking from the audience. We can feel, if not explain, whether tension changes and shape changes are congruent or disparate.

Let us look once more at Leonardo's "Madonna and Child with St. Anne" (Figure 3). St. Anne's left arm is widening at the shoulder, but the tension-flow in her arm is bound and even. It looks as if she is holding her breath and emphasizing her right arm to get more space for herself than for her daughter. But mother and daughter do harmonize in their facial expressions, as their lips quiver at the angles and widen. This implies generosity and adaptability, and gives the appearance of benevolence. However, there are more clashes and contrasts between them in other areas. As Mary shortens in the middle, bending towards her child, her mother's figure remains erect, and there is considerable lengthening in her right neck and shoulder area. She watches what her daughter is doing, but she is neither participating nor supporting her. She seems to want to emphasize that she is the bigger or taller of the two.

This contrast of big versus small, combined with Anne's wideness and the narrowing of Mary's arms, suggests that St. Anne has greater esteem for herself than for her daughter. It might be that Mary represents Leonardo's mother, while Anne symbolizes his older, aristocratic stepmother. There are many contrasting features, and they cannot all be mentioned here; they also extend to the relationship between Mary and the Christ Child. Mary bulges out of her mother's lap; it seems that she would like to fill herself with the baby she is reaching for. The baby and the lamb show contradictory shapes; their heads bulge towards Mary, while the child's arm turns away and grasps the lamb, which is pulling away from him. Their unity, however, is shown in the extension of Mary's arms to the child's arms and to the torso and tail of the animal, perhaps little Jesus' transitional object.

In the shape-flow of these three figures we are seeing the narcissistic and anaclitic core of the three generations. The proud and aloof grandmother, the mother longing for her child, and the child ambivalently veering between his mother and the transitional object, representing the mother he loved and perhaps lost. To get more insight into the constant relationships of the two adults and the budding constancy of the child, we turn to more advanced patterns of shaping.

The Shaping of Space

Through shape flow, we express our capacity for self- and other-relatedness. Through shaping of space coupled with efforts, we express relationships to others who are permanently represented intrapsychically. Shaping is a term coined by Lamb (1965), defined in our study as the individual's linear and multi-dimensional alterations of the shape of the space around them.

By **shaping in directions** — moving **across** the body, **sideways**, **upward**, **downward**, **forward** or **backward** — we reach into linear space and locate various points in it. This enables us to localize others in relation to ourselves and represents the simplest way of differentiating ourselves from other people in fairly specific ways: reaching for them, moving away from them, or ignoring them by looking elsewhere.

St. Anne looks down with a benevolent smile. From this

high vantage point, she seems condescending (Figure 3). Mary moves downward and forward towards her child, while the child turns sideways and looks up toward Mary's face. The lamb looks at her, as well, by raising his head towards her. These directions localize a common point in space. There is only one line between the mother's, the child's and the lamb's eyes, and this line also points toward the grandmother's eyes. However, her eyes are unreceptive, as they pursue their own line of vision, perpendicular and at a sharp angle to the oblique line of vision of the others.

Shaping in planes is multidimensional, representing the complex nature of constant relationships. It goes beyond linear connection to express interactions in three dimensions, the horizontal, vertical and sagittal planes. Open shaping exposes the body to the space around it: **spreading** in the horizontal plane, **ascending** in the vertical plane, and **advancing** in the saggital plane. These movements indicate accessibility to contact (spreading), seeking of ideals or idealizing of objects (ascending), and desire to make contact with others (advancing). Closed shaping involves **enclosing** in the horizontal plane, **descending** in the vertical plane, and **retreating** in the saggital plane. These movements signify limitation of contact (enclosing), teaching or explaining (descending), and wanting to be left alone (retreating).

Mary's spatial shaping is multi-dimensional, indicating the complexity of her relationship to her child. In contrast, her mother's lack of shaping in planes makes her comparable to the background rocks and the immovable tree that stands erect and inanimate behind her. Mary advances fully towards her child; she grasps him, but does not pull him up. Her pelvis spreads horizontally, as if she was trying to make room for him. He spreads as much as he can, using his head alone, and ascends toward his mother. They have some reciprocal communication horizontally, the plane of human contact. Since the mother's right arm is descending and the child is attempting to ascend, one would expect them to meet, but the child turns away by enclosing the lamb's neck with his arm, and holding on tightly. With his body and limbs he advances toward the lamb, mirroring his mother's advance toward him. The mother's descending movement harmonizes with the strength that emanates from her spreading pelvis. The child approaches the lamb hesitantly, with rudimentary strength. The mother's constancy in relation to gravity is evident, in the harmony expressed between strength and descending. From this constancy arises an acceptance of different qualities in mother and child; weighing each other's determination becomes the source of evaluation and understanding.

Mary's deceleration, as she advances toward the child with her whole body, shows her constancy in time. The child turns his head towards her, but with the rest of his body he advances toward the lamb. The lamb also displays conflict; he seems to advance toward the mother and child with his head, but the rest of his body seems to retreat. The mother's deceleration softens the strength that radiates from her pelvis. In a loving way, she is ready to wait, but she is determined that eventually there will be a reunion with the Child.

Through this example, we become aware that in appraising various aspects of body shape and shaping in space, we have immersed ourselves in an appraisal of the self and the object as revealed in the visual arts. The dynamic interplay of forces through effort provides the content; for instance, we learn that the mother is strong, but loving and accommodating, while the grandmother is aloof. The mother's relationship to the child becomes comprehensive when it is structured by the open attitudes of spreading and advancing that mitigate her descent upon the child. The grandmother's narcissistic stance, and the child's conflicted relationships, contrast with the mother's attempt to be reunited with her child.

We see that Leonardo reproduces the mother image that he yearns for, and depicts his grandmother or stepmother as genteel, but also aloof and hard. He shows himself veering between his desire for reunion with his mother, and his love for his transitional object, a vestige of the mother of his early infancy.

Expressive Art and Primary Prevention

Primary prevention aims to optimize development, to remove obstacles to developmental progression, and to strengthen the child's resources for coping with ordinary stressors. Why and how do we use the arts for prevention? It is well known that artistic activity provides outlets for impulses and desires that are then deflected from their original aim. We will not allow children to put a pencil in their mouth, but we will encourage them to insert a flute in the same place. This process of sublimation is the mainstay of creativity and cultural achievement. De-aggressivization (Hartmann, 1939/ 1958) helps to convert hostile impulses into achievement. We let children pound a piece of clay rather than our furniture; in so doing, they change the form of the object which is being manipulated (Kestenberg, 1990).

In all these examples, the little artist is a performer, and uses deflected aggressive and erotic impulses to change the nature of the original artistic material through paint, body movement, or music (Kestenberg, 1990). By looking at art or dance and listening or moving to music, the child becomes an appreciative audience who can vicariously enjoy the creativity and performances of others. As watchers and as listeners, children derive inspiration for their own creations, as well as skills to improve their own performances.

In one of our activities at the Center for Parents and Children (which operated between 1972 and 1990), we presented young children (18 months to 4 years) with postcard reproductions of great paintings. These were placed on small easels at their eye level while they worked with crayons or paints. We did not tell them to copy or look at the paintings, but our results show that they were greatly influenced by what they saw. Not only did they emulate colors and shapes, but they also changed their composition according to their perception of the picture before them. Once children learned to create while viewing, they could create without copying. The internalization of a picture, a dance or a song provided them with images to use, and elaborate on, in the formation of internal objects. They re-externalized these images to reinforce the memory of absent people:

• Minnie (15 months) could fall asleep easier when a picture of her mother and herself was hung in her crib.

• Johnny (18 months) held on to a roughly drawn picture

of his mother when she had to leave him at the Center for several hours.

• Tony (2-1/2 years) awoke from anesthesia after an operation and began to sing the Center songs to remind him of the atmosphere and the people at the Center, who had prepared him for the operation.

All along, I am speaking here of infants and toddlers as creative artists, without engaging in the controversy about the elements of "real art" (Gardner, 1980). From the beginning, infants create new objects out of the matrix of their developmental stance and out of current inner and outer stimuli. Winnicott traced this creativity from the stage

> at which the integrating tendencies of the infant bring about a state in which the infant is a unit, a whole person, with an inside and an outside, and a person living in the body, and more or less bounded by skin. Once outside means 'not-Me,' then inside means 'Me,' there is now a place in which to store things . . . . The child is now not only a potential creator of the world, but also the child becomes capable to populate the world with samples of his or her own inner life. So gradually the child is able to 'cover' almost any external event, and perception is almost synonymous with creation (1953, p. 91).

Winnicott discovered the world of transitional objects and phenomena, and he described the intermediate area between the mother and child as the space from which creativity arises. The lamb in Leonardo's painting may be a transitional object representing part of the child and part of the mother, but he is not placed between them. Here the child is torn between what he perceives as his mother's longing for him, and the lamb's resistance to following him wherever he wants to go. The conflict between wanting to be with mother and with the transitional object, which represents the mother as she once

Figure 4.

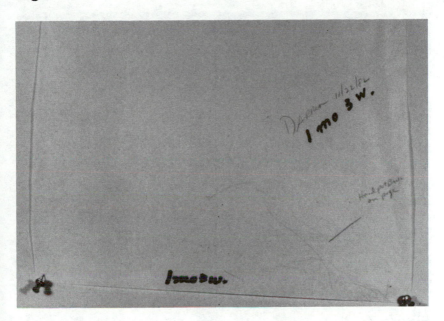

Figure 5.

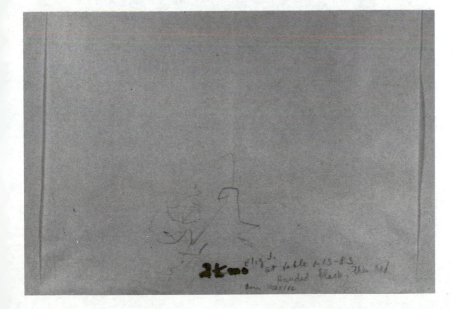

Figure 6.

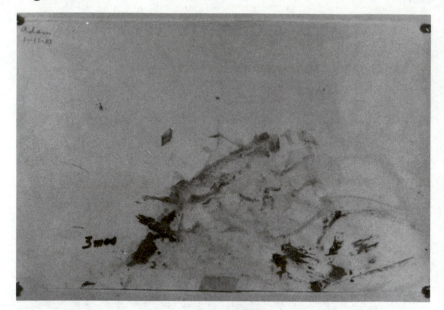

Figure 7.

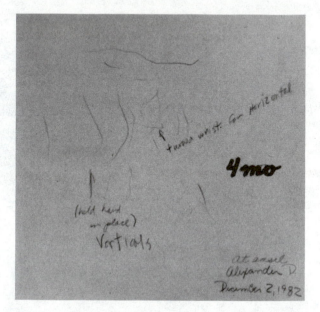

was, is presented. The lamb itself is torn between the mother and the child. The mother is inviting and giving, and the lamb looks up to her, but also balks at the same time. The child not only creates the mother the way he sees her or wants to see her, but also creates an image of the way he saw her in the past. The resistance of the lamb may depict the fact that Leonardo's mother did not follow him when he was taken away from her.

I once suggested to Winnicott that creativity cannot emanate from the intermediate zone between mother and child, although it may emerge there. All creativity comes from inside and radiates outward, enveloping the outside and the inside of the object, as well as the self. Thus all art is concerned with the creation and re-creation of objects and the self as they are now, and as they are remembered from the past.

The Use of Art to Promote Development

Even very young babies identify objects in terms of their motion and location. At first their eyes follow their mother's voice or footsteps. When they grow older, they search for their mother's face where it disappeared from their view. By six weeks, many babies imitate finger movement. The six-month old listens to music and vocalizes rhythmically (Papousek & Papousek, 1981). A baby with a grasp reflex will hold a pencil, and will leave pencil marks on a surface that his hand is held close to, but will have no awareness of having left an image there. By three months, some babies will look at the image, especially if it is red, and by six months some babies are able to connect the image with their activities. Their productions are disconnected lines of varying lengths (Figure 4), traces of their centripetal and centrifugal motions, and horizontal motions that are parallel to the body.

Young infants attune to maternal tension changes as the mother attunes to theirs. As they breathe with her, it helps them to regulate their shape-flow. Their imitations of her facial expressions regulate their mimetics. In this process, they create images of their body and their mother's body, images based on sameness. From the start, baby and mother come together and separate, allowing the infant to develop a feeling for what is "me" and what is "not-me." Lifton (1979) speaks of "centering" the experience of the self along three dimensions, one of which is the dimension of space. He believes that adult imagery flows out of the imagery built up during childhood, but is continuously transformed by the inner re-creation of new experiences. What Lifton metaphorically calls the spatial plane is the first structuring of relationships that really occurs in the horizontal, feeding plane (Laban, 1960). In this plane, we develop our sense of self as expanding and shrinking in relation to the expanding and shrinking body of the mother. In this plane, the body image of the infant is created from multisensory experiences (Schilder, 1935/1950; Kestenberg, 1983). This begins when we learn to turn to the breast and grasp. The subsequent image formations and re-formations in this and the two other planes can be considered the internal prototype of the arts. Once the child becomes capable of creating or performing, the image is projected outward onto the artistic medium.

Rhythm — which is intrinsic to all living tissue and to visual art, dance and music — repeats patterns, thus bridging the discontinuity of experience. Cessation of rhythm brings on purposeful, bi-phasic or tri-phasic actions, such as reaching for an object and grasping it, then bringing it to the mouth. Efforts and shaping of space develop and mature within the sphere of these purposive activities. These activities control the rhythms of tension- and shape-flow, and can create their own rhythms. The self and the narcissistic object evolve from feelings based on tension-flow and structured by shape-flow; the constant object has its motorical origin in the dynamics of effort, structured by shaping. Each re-formation of an early experience revolves around the early self and the early object, and thus abounds in the rhythmic components of tension- and shape-flow. By its re-organization through effort and shape, a new bounded object is created. Each re-formation of an experience, and its integration with the present and the future, re-creates the objects of the past and brings them in accord with the representation of present objects.

Through the union of feeling, self, and object, there evolves

Figure 8.

Figure 9.

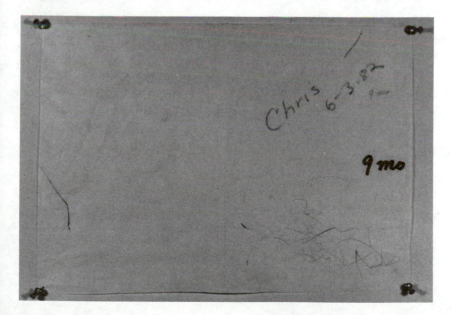

Figure 10.

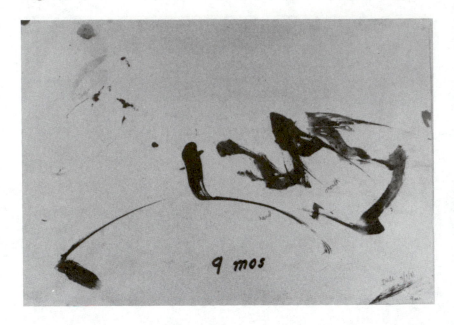

Figure 11.

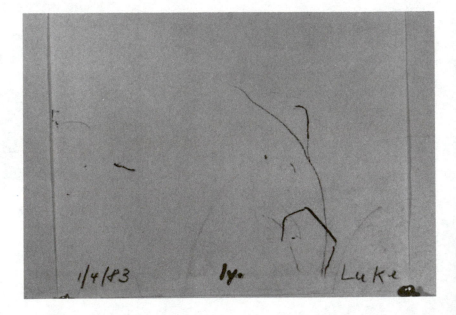

a center of the self- and object-representation. Once established, these representations are in continuous flux, but the flux persists against a background of stable, unchangeable images. As relationships change, the form of the object changes, but the core-form remains the same.

In the oral phase, in which the nutritional sucking and biting rhythms predominate, the child builds a self-image as a nursling, and an image of the parent as the feeding mother. The baby mirrors her face, and approximates her facial expressions, communing with her as a precursor to communication (Kestenberg et al, 1971). By singing or speaking to her baby in a sing-song voice (Stern, 1977), by allowing the infant to build a visual image of her face and mirror it, the mother helps her child acquire tools for multi-sensory object building. When we ask the mother to hold the baby's hand that holds the pencil, and allow it to move over the paper, she helps her child to leave a permanent trace of these attempts to build the object and the self (Figures 4, 5, 6, 7, & 8).

Once children gain control over the horizontal plane, they begin to draw lines purposively. They recognize that what they see is the result of their action. While their early lines are fragmented, in the second half of their first year their lines become longer and more vertical, rather than mostly horizontal, curved and looping like their earlier lines (Figures 9, 10, 11).

In the anal phase, the child's orientation shifts to focus on conquering gravity, which will become the content of adult life. At this age, children are not just "in love with the world" (Greenacre, 1957; Mahler, Pine & Bergmann 1975). They seem to be infatuated with the vertical plane, in which transactions with gravity occur. We can witness the birth of dance when toddlers kneel or hold on to stand, bending their knees and straightening them to music, using an anal twisting or straining rhythm. We observe their muscular activity becoming more forceful and intense, and their voices deepening. Soon they will climb and try to jump, but it will take some time before they can get both feet safely off the ground. These dancing toddlers, going up and down in delight, are creating their first dance step, one which mimics being tossed up in the air and

Figure 12.

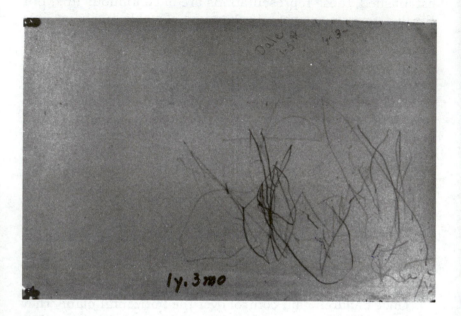

1y. 3mo

Figure 13.

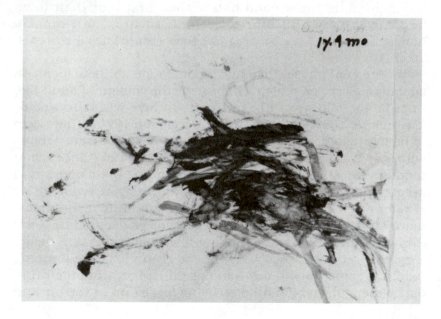

1y. 4mo

caught by their parents. The dance becomes an illusion of flying through the air, reaching up to the height of their parents, and then falling back down to their own earthbound position.

At 14 months, children begin to draw continuously. It seems that they cannot stop making rhythmical loops on paper (Figures 12, 13). Some walking toddlers will no longer draw while sitting at a table; they must stand while drawing. Those who do sit, draw increasingly vertical lines (Figure 14). Towards the end of their second year, when they become aware of the density in their bellies, and lean a lot against the maternal belly, the center of their pictures becomes dense, thick, and prominent (Figures 14, 15, 16). They begin to isolate some circles, but their circles continue to flow into each other, since they cannot stop their rhythmic activity to effect closure (Figure 17). In their productions we recognise the vestiges of the oral object and of the feeding mother with whom they overlap. Although proud possessors of a middle, they still share their center of gravity with their mother. Their constancy of weight is now developing; Lifton apparently refers to this experience in describing a centering of the self "that discriminates emotional values between various images of the self" (1979). Toddlers feel their weight as heavy or light, and feel their own budding strength compared to the strength of their parents. They practice this centering in the vertical plane, contrasting strength with the lightness of soaring. In this plane, they learn to appraise and evaluate by looking up and down, and by ascending and descending, which they coordinate with feelings of differential weight. They are becoming intentional and determined, accepting things as good or rejecting them as bad, until they learn to accept both qualities in themselves and in their objects.

In the third year, the urethral phase, time becomes of the essence. It is then that music becomes a symbolic expression of feelings more than ever before. Children can sing tunes and compose music; time sequences can be anticipated and become meaningful. At the end of this phase, children not only initiate songs, but know when they end, so their singing becomes less repetitive. Their self-images of climbing and standing are now superceded by images of running. Their

Figure 14.

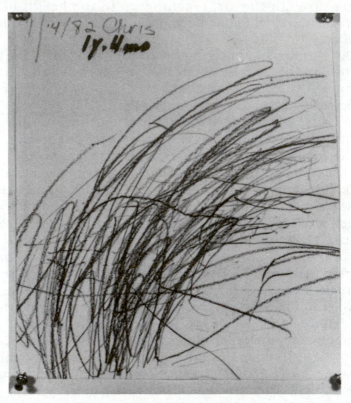

Figure 15.

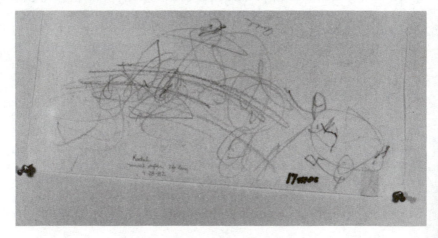

Figure 16.

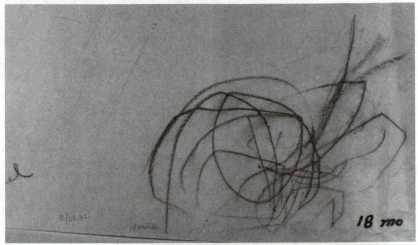

Figure 17.

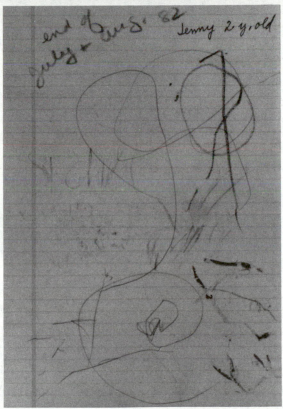

Figure 18.

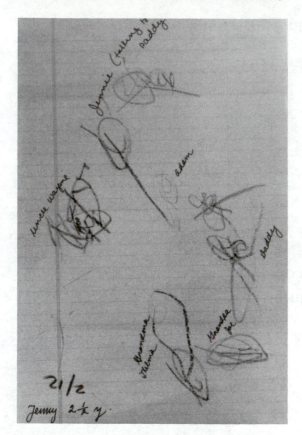

Figure 19.

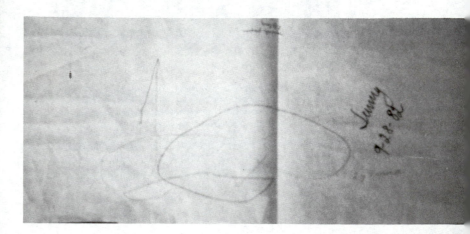

Figure 20.

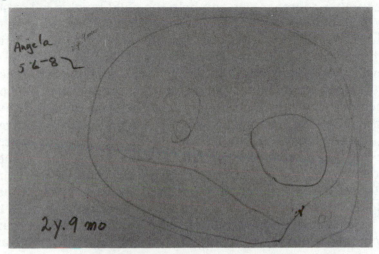

Figure 21.

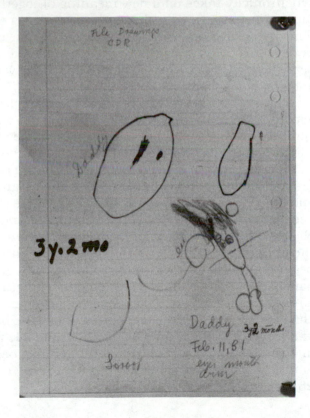

images of the training mother are now superseded by images of a containing mother who can help the child break a fall or stop the flow of urine (Figure 17). Lifton speaks of centering on the temporal plane by "using older images and shapes in ways that can anticipate . . . future events" (1979). This type of centering develops in the urethral phase; at this time children practise getting ahead or lagging behind in time on the sagittal plane. They can now start dancing to music and stop when the music stops. They can hear a story without asking that it be read over again. The large and small loops which had been criss-crossed by vertical lines in the preceding phase are becoming more directed, and the middle of the picture is becoming more fluid (Figures 16, 17). Eventually, closed forms begin to appear (Figure 18), and drawings appear to be going places (Figure 17). At the same time, their dancing becomes more clearly locomotor, dancing to music helps to regulate time, and synchronicity takes on a new meaning of togetherness, rather than sameness. In this phase, the rudiments of constancy in time are created and even "yesterday" or "later" can be depicted in drawings. However, the newly-created self and object still bear the traces of earlier objects, and earlier ways of drawing, dancing and vocalizing do re-appear.

Three-year olds integrate all of their previous objects and accomplishments into their preoccupation with their inner genital organs (Kestenberg, 1982). The three dimensions in which object ties have been structured become amalgamated. In their pictures, a three-dimensional space is created, with a distinct inside. Circles have smaller circles and loops inside, and the face encompasses the body as a whole (Figures 19, 20). Feelings radiate from inside out to animate and vitalize all the objects in the outside world. Each object becomes a baby, while the child plays the role of the mother. At this age, children begin making up songs, composed from bits of melodies, and dancing out song stories. Through dance, pictures and music, a new being is created, a baby that no longer exists because the child is now "big." At the end of this phase the baby "grows up" and a picture of a child emerges (Figures 21, 22). The visual image in the next phase, the outer genital, beginning at age four, is not only complete, but has an activity content (Figures 23, 24).

Rather than sketch out how object- and self-building proceeds in further development, let me stop here to say a few words about helping children to build and re-build significant images through art. We use all media, and do not forget that all of them are tools for object building, even in the earliest phases.

Throughout development, objects (including the self as an object) are built, lost and re-built. This is a continuously revolving process: things which leave our personal space are lost, and people that soar to unknown heights or disappear into the horizon are also lost. Remembering them, internalizing their images, children revive them, and with each new loss and recovery, new features are added to the image. This building and re-building process has a rhythmic character, against a background of permanent images. An image does not have the same vitality, elasticity or plasticity as a living being. The more the image can be endowed with living characteristics, the more real it seems, even in memory. When we recall the mother of our childhood, the image is shadowy until we begin to paint her portrait in our mind; until we remember her voice, the songs she sang, how she walked and danced, how she smelled, and the smoothness of her skin. Artists may have a particularly well-developed capacity to reproduce the image of a living person, a person that no longer exists in the same way. If we recall ourselves as children, we have an even harder time recreating the baby that lingers inside us. However, we can create a baby by drawing or painting it, or we can act out being a baby, giving it vocalizations and rhythmic motions, until it seems to be real in the here and now.

By providing babies and toddlers with repeated experiences of picture-building, by evoking vocalization and introducing them to music, dance and singing, we provide them with enriched means to build their self- and object-images. When young babies are seated at a piano on someone's lap, they feel the movement of the person who is holding them, playing and singing. We let three-month-olds feel the impact of their movement on a hard surface, and eventually help them see that their motions have created a sound. By giving young children daily opportunities to dance, we enhance their capacity to deal with space, weight and time within an optimal

Figure 22.

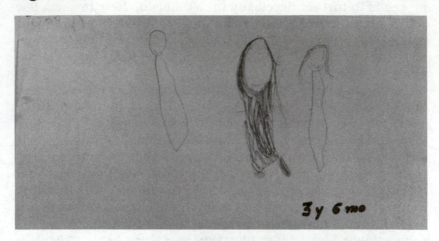

Figure 23.

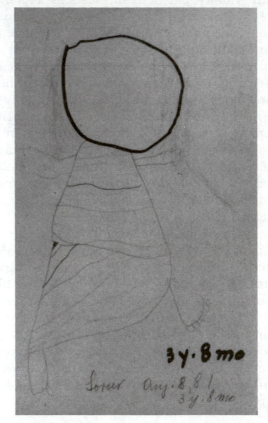

Figure 24.

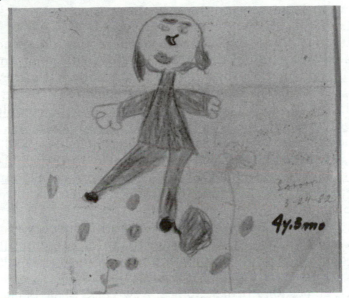

structure to experience all three spatial planes. As they leave the oral phase, we help them to recreate the oral mother, using all media, and to build the anal training and later the urethral containing mother as enduring images. We help them to develop their maternal potential and create a new image out of the earlier ones, one which distinguishes between mother and child, and yet unites them through reproduction.

Lastly, we must stress that it is not only the experience of creation through performing that must be introduced early in life, but also the experience of observing works of art, dance, and music. These experiences help in elaborating self- and object-images through identification with another person's creation. Through participation and internalization, the watcher, the motionless dancer, and the listener extract what is needed for inspiration and for making all imagery more beautiful, more vital, and more enduring.

References

Arnheim, R. (1969). Visual thinking. Berkeley, CA: University of California Press.

Freud, A. (1965). Normality and pathology in childhood: Assessments of development. In The writings of Anna Freud (Vol. 6). New York: International Universities Press.

Freud, S. (1953). The interpretation of dreams. In J. Strachey (Ed. and Trans.), The standard edition of the complete psychological works of Sigmund Freud (Vols. 4 - 5). London: Hogarth Press. (Original work published 1900)

Freud, S. (1955). The Moses of Michaelangelo. In The standard edition of the complete psychological works of Sigmund Freud (Vol. 13). London: Hogarth Press. (Original work published 1914)

Freud, S. (1957). Leonardo da Vinci and a memory of his childhood. In The standard edition of the complete psychological works of Sigmund Freud (Vol. 11). London: Hogarth Press. (Original work published 1910)

Gardner, H. (1980). Artful scribbles. New York: Basic Books.

Greenacre, P. (1957). The childhood of the artist: Libidinal phase development and giftedness. In The psychoanalytic study of the child (Vol. 12). New York: International Universities Press.

Hartmann, H. (1958). Ego psychology and the problem of adaptation. New York: International Universities Press. (Original work published 1939)

Kestenberg, J. S. (1975). From organ-object imagery to self and object representations. In Children and parents: Psychoanalytic studies in development. New York: Jason Aronson.

Kestenberg, J. S. (1977). The role of movement patterns in development (Vol. 1). New York: Dance Notation Bureau Press.

Kestenberg, J. S. (1982). The inner-genital phase, pre-phallic and pre-oedipal. In D. Mendell (Ed.), Early female development. New York: Spectrum Publications.

Kestenberg, J. S. (1985). The role of movement patterns in diagnosis and prevention. In Shaskan & Parker (Eds.), Papers in honor of Paul Schilder. New York: Columbia University Press.

Kestenberg, J. S. (1990). The multiple facets of work: A developmental study. In P. Lewis & S. Loman (Eds.), The Kestenberg movement profile: Its past, present applications and future directions. Keene, NH: Antioch New England Graduate School.

Kestenberg, J. S. & Buelte, A. (1977). Prevention, infant therapy, and the treatment of adults: I. Toward understanding mutuality. International Journal of Psychoanalytic Psychotherapy, 6, 339-366.

Kestenberg, J. S. & Buelte, A. (1977). Prevention, infant therapy, and the treatment of adults: II. Mutual holding and holding oneself up. International Journal of Psychoanalytic Psychotherapy, 6, 367-396.

Kestenberg, J. S. & Buelte, A. (1983). Prevention, infant therapy, and the treatment of adults: III. In J. Call & E. Galenson (Eds.), Frontiers in infant psychiatry. New York: Basic Books.

Kestenberg, J. S., Marcus, H., Robbins, E., Berlowe, J., & Buelte, A. (1975). Development of the young child as expressed through bodily movement: I. In Children and parents: Psychoanalytic studies in development. New York: Jason Aronson.

Kestenberg, J. S. & Sossin, M. (1979). The role of movement patterns in development (Vol. 2). New York: Dance Notation Bureau Press.

Kris, E. (1952). Psychoanalytic explorations in art. New York: International Universities Press.

Laban, R. (1920). Die Welt des Taenzers (The world of the dancer). Stuttgart: Walter Siefert.

Laban, R. (1935). Ein Leben fuer den Tanz (A life for dance). Dresden: Carl Reibner.

Laban, R. (1960). Effort: Economy in body movement (2nd ed.). London: MacDonald & Evans.

Laban, R. (1971). Dance as a discipline. In L. Ullmann (Ed.) Rudolf Laban speaks about movement and dance (p. 22). Woburn Hill, Surrey: Laban Art of Movement Centre.

Laban, R. (1971). Dance in general. In L. Ullmann (Ed.) Rudolf Laban speaks about movement and dance (p. 56). Woburn Hill, Surrey: Laban Art of Movement Centre.

Lamb, W. (1965). Posture and gesture. London: Gerald

Duckworth.

Langer, S. K. (1953). Feeling and form. New York: Charles Scribner.

Lifton, R. J. (1983). The broken connection. New York: Basic Books.

Mahler, M. S., Pine, F., & Bergmann, A. (1975). The psychological birth of the infant. New York: Basic Books.

Ostwald, P. F. (1963). Soundmaking: The acoustic communication of emotion. Springfield, IL: Charles C. Thomas.

Papousek, M. & Papousek, H. (1981). Musical elements in the infant's vocalization: Their significance for communication, cognition and creativity. In L. P. Lipsitt (Ed.), Advances in infancy research (Vol. 1, pp.163-224). Norwood, NJ: Ablex Publishing.

Schilder, P. (1950). Image and appearance of the human body. New York: International Universities Press. (Original work published 1935)

Shields, A. & Robbins, A. (1980). Music in expressive therapy. In A. Robbins (Ed.), Expressive therapy. New York: Human Sciences Press.

Stern, D. (1977). The first relationship: infant and mother. Cambridge, MA: Harvard University Press.

Winnicott, D. W. (1953). Transitional objects and transitional phenomena. International Journal of Psychoanalysis, 34, 89-97.

Notes

[1]Presented at the 2nd Annual Leonard Strahl Memorial Lecture at the Institute for Expressive Analysis, Pratt Creative Arts Therapy Department, 1983. In an abbreviated form, this paper was also given (with Susan Loman and Carol Fishman) in a workshop at the New England Council of Creative Therapies Conference, Brown University, R.I., 1979.

[2]From the Center for Parents and Children, sponsored by Child Development Research, Sands Point, New York.

[3]For a systematic presentation of movement patterns, see Kestenberg and Sossin, 1979. For a detailed description of inner genitality, see Kestenberg, 1982.

Fetal Movement Notation: A Method of Attuning to the Fetus

Susan Loman, M.A., A.D.T.R.

Introduction

This paper presents a clinical application of the Kestenberg Movement Profile, a system of movement notation and analysis developed by Judith S. Kestenberg, M.D. (Kestenberg & Sossin, 1979) and the Sands Point Movement Study Group (Kestenberg, Marcus, Robbins et al, 1975). Kestenberg began developing the profile in 1952, in an attempt to devise a form of movement notation to record the nonverbal expressions of mothers and infants. She collaborated with the Sands Point Movement Study Group, Irmgard Bartenieff (Bartenieff & Lewis, 1980), and Warren Lamb (1965). By 1965 the profile had been extended beyond Kestenberg's original objective to assess individuals of all ages. The KMP's interpretive framework is based on Anna Freud's metapsychological profile (1965), reflecting Kestenberg's psychoanalytic orientation.

Child Development Research, a non-profit organization for research and training with children and families, has sponsored two programs to apply Kestenberg's movement studies to families. The Center for Parents and Children opened in 1972, with the goal of preventing emotional disorders in young children. The Prenatal Project was also founded in the early 1970's to train prospective parents and obstetric nurses to become aware of the preferred rhythms of the fetus and newborn, and to respond in a similar rhythm in order to facilitate early mother-child bonding (Kestenberg, 1975).

This paper will present the work of the Prenatal Project: its goals, methods (training classes) and some of its preliminary results. The key concept of attunement, or nonverbal empathy, will be described as the basis of both fetal movement notation patterns will also be presented. Finally, suggestions for further research and application of fetal movement notation will be discussed.

Preparation For The Child Training

The Prenatal Project was designed by Kestenberg and colleagues to help expectant parents prepare for the arrival of the new baby. These "Preparation for the Child" classes differ from other pregnancy classes in that they not only prepare the parents for the birth process, but also for the initial development of the relationship between parent and child (Kestenberg, 1980). In this class, the parents are given the opportunity to re-discover the movement patterns of babies, which differ a great deal from adult movement patterns. They are encouraged to develop an image of how the unborn child moves, and are taught to notate the tension changes in fetal movement. Kestenberg describes the results of this training process:

> This [training] not only brought them into a type of communication with the fetus, but it taught them to consider the fetus as a partner, an idea which then pervaded their deliveries. They were aware of the fetal movement during labor and had a feeling of continuity from inside to the outside by observing the movement of the baby as soon as it was born. The expectation that one can recognize the baby by the way it had moved inside of the mother strengthened the feeling of belonging mothers develop after the initial estrangement from the infant (1980, p. 59).

In these classes, the expectant mother is encouraged to keep a journal of her fetal movement notations, physical sensations, feelings and dreams. Kestenberg believes that many dreams during pregnancy are related to fetal movement (1982), with specific themes according to the stage of pregnancy (1976). For example, dreams in the third trimester often have mobile themes involving flowing water or riding in vehicles such as sleds and watermobiles.

Special exercises are taught to help the expectant mother's body actively stretch and adjust to the fetus. These exercises emphasize the growing movements of widening, lengthening and bulging, helping to make room for the fetus and to avoid pain from pressure on the bladder or back. The mother is taught to breathe into painful spots, which also encourages stretching to accommodate the baby's expansion. A modified form of belly dancing is taught to increase flexibility and coordination, aiding in a smooth delivery. This process of adjusting the expectant mother's alignment to accommodate the additional weight of pregnancy helps to give her the feeling that she is actively carrying the baby, instead of being pulled down by it (Loman, 1980). Another benefit for expectant mothers is an improved body image, at a time when many women may be feeling awkward about their growing size. One participant describes this aspect of the program:

> [The exercises] helped us to stay in shape and cope with the increase in body weight . . . Common problems such as heartburn and excesssive urinary frequency were helped with posture changes so that the weight was shifted from the bladder or stomach. Simple things like — How do you get up off the floor or chair? . . . What is the best way to rest with your legs elevated? — proved to be very helpful (Jordan, 1981).

The prenatal classes have been experimenting with introducing the fetus to music, through headphones placed on the mother's abdomen (Kestenberg, 1982). The idea of this exercise is that music which they hear in the womb may be especially soothing to them after birth. Results so far indicate that the fetus responds to the music either by becoming more still (perhaps sleeping) or by moving more actively — and some mothers are reporting that after birth their babies continue to respond to the music which was played in the womb. It should be noted, however, that the fetus has no choice in the selection of the music, and more research is needed to differentiate negative responses (music too loud or unpleasant to the baby) from positive responses (music enjoyed by the baby).

Another kind of musical expression is also used in the class — the expectant mother is taught to sing deep tones to accompany labor and pushing contractions. These vocalizations are practiced throughout the pregnancy. They have been shown to be effective in increasing the dilation of the cervix during the transition phase of delivery, and in enabling the expectant mother to actively engage during labor, instead of distracting herself from the pain.

In several instances, Kestenberg has attended deliveries as a coach, and videotaped the birth process. These videotapes reveal how mothers utilize the concepts learned in the "Preparation for the Child" classes. As one mother writes,

> . . . I notated my child's fetal movements and drew pictures of what I thought it looked like inside. I put headphones on my stomach and played rock music to this baby. I even talked to this unborn child of mine and so did my son, Keith — "Hello baby!" he would scream into my stomach . . . Dr. Kestenberg's presence during my labor and delivery was a wonderful and extremely helpful experience. [She] moaned, groaned, pushed and even screamed with me (Amoruso, 1982, p.4).[1]

Attunement

Attunement, or nonverbal empathy, is the basis of fetal movement notation, the notation of tension-flow movement patterns, and the early parent-child bonding process. Therefore, it is important to understand the basic premise of attunement and its variations.

One form of attunement is **complete attunement**, which can be found in the mother-infant relationship. Kestenberg explains that "complete attunement is based on mutual empathy or on excessive similarity between partners. There is not only a sameness of needs and responses, but also a synchronization in rhythms" (1975, p. 161). She postulates that needs and feelings are reflected in changes in muscular tension (**tension-flow**). In **tension flow attunement** — whether between mother and child, between adults, between children, or among groups — needs and feelings are responsively duplicated on the level of physical sensation. In **complete attunement of tension-flow,** which can be found between mother and nursing child, there is a kinesthetic identification in which the muscular tensions of one are simultaneously felt in the other's body (see below for a more in-depth discussion of tension-flow). However, this duplication of the flow of muscular tension does not necessarily require duplication of body shape (Loman, 1988).

Visual attunement and **touch attunement** involve the same principle of duplication response, but are perceived and expressed through other forms of contact. Visual attunement is accomplished by observing the level and rhythm of tension in another person's moving body, and then matching that tension-rhythm in one's own body. Again, the muscular tension alone is duplicated, not the shape of the body. For example, to attune to an infant who is vigorously kicking its legs, one could move in rhythm with the kicking with any body part, matching the muscular tension, rhythmicity, and speed of the baby's movements.

Touch attunement is similar to visual attunement, based on touch contact: for example, hold hands and respond to any changes in the other person's position, pressure or rhythm with changes in hand movements (touching). As in other forms of attunement, the responses occur simultaneously with the perception of movement, without delay. Even the smallest changes, such as the contraction or stretch of muscles, will be duplicated. However, the size of the attuning response does not have to reflect the size of the original movement; the response to a tiny muscular stretch could be felt in the responder's whole hand or throughout their entire body.

Attunement is very similar to the approach used by Marian Chace, a founder of dance therapy, in working with psychiatric patients. Chace describes her technique of making initial contact with a patient:

> The movements used in establishing initial
> contact with a patient may be qualitatively
> similar to those of the patient (not an exact
> mimicking since this is often construed by the
> patient as mocking) . . . The following is an
> example of how the patient's muscular tensions
> are picked up by the therapist and carried into
> dance action. One patient stands hunched
> forward, contracted through the abdomen, his
> whole posture that of a person in terror. The
> therapist feels the tension within her own
> abdomen, and using this as a center of action,
> she develops a tension relaxation dance
> sequence (1975, p. 73).

Parents are first taught to perceive fetal movement with touch attunement exercises. They learn to become sensitive to movement changes which they can feel but cannot see (such as intrauterine fetal movements). In one exercise, the expectant mother's partner gives her a back massage with a variety of tension-flow patterns (i.e., rhythms and attributes, see below). This rhythmic massage provides sensations similar to the flutters and pushes of the fetus. She attunes to these sensations by duplicating them with hand movements, simultaneously tensing and relaxing her arms and hands. After learning these exercises, she is taught tension-flow notation to record her perceptions of fetal tension changes. This tension-flow writing tracks the rhythm of the fetus' muscular contractions and releases along a time axis, producing tracings which look like EKG recordings. Before this notation is described further, however, the KMP's concept of tension-flow must be defined in more depth.

Tension-Flow

According to the KMP, **tension-flow** is a manifestation of animate muscle elasticity, reflecting the continual rhythmic variation between the polarities of **bound flow** and **free flow** in muscular tissue (Sossin & Loman, 1982). Fetal movement

Figure 1. Tension Flow Rhythms

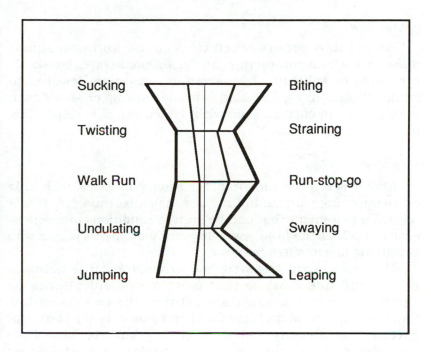

Figure 2. Tension Flow Attributes

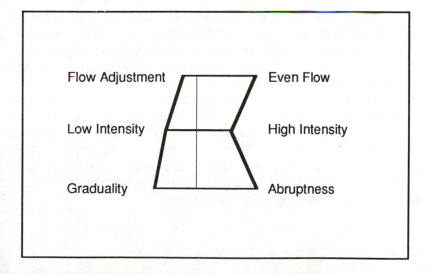

notation is based on the polarity between bound flow and free flow.

Bound Flow

Bound flow occurs when the agonist and antagonist muscles are both contracting, as during isometric exercises. It restrains or inhibits the movement impulse, leading to immobilization or rigidity, and is needed to stop or slow down. Bound flow can often be seen when an individual is responding to a dangerous situation.

Free Flow

Free flow is a contraction of the agonist muscles, with little or no opposing contraction of the antagonist muscles. It is a releasing movement that can be seen in conditions of safety or ease — such as the fluid, swinging arm movements of one who is walking in a carefree manner.

Healthy functioning strikes a dynamic balance between bound and free flow, so that most movement alternates rhythmically on a continuum between the two polarities. Variations in bound and free flow can be described in terms of rhythm and intensity. Ten different rhythms (**tension-flow rhythms**) and six intensity factors (**tension-flow attributes**) are catalogued in the KMP (Kestenberg and Sossin, 1979).

Tension-Flow Rhythms

Tension flow rhythms are periodic alternations between bound and free flow in ten developmentally based patterns: sucking, biting, twisting, straining, running, stopping/starting, undulating, swaying, jumping and leaping. Although they are developmentally based, all ten rhythms are potentially available to the fetus. In interpretation, specific tension-flow rhythms are connected with particular modes of drive discharge and need satisfaction. An individual's preferred manner of dealing with drives and needs is reflected in their predominant tension-flow rhythms (Figure 1). When two or more individuals share similar tension-flow rhythms, the core of empathic communication is present.

Tension-Flow Attributes

Tension-flow attributes describe tension-flow changes in terms of six qualities of intensity, which determine the expression of affect. They also reflect an individual's temperament and characteristics of arousal or quiescence (Sossin & Loman, 1982).

1. Even flow

Tension is stabilized at the same level; indicates ease, resting, steadiness, steadfastness and an even temperament.

2. Flow adjustment

Tension adjusts itself and adapts to meet new situations; indicates an accommodating temperament.

3. High intensity

Tension reaches extreme bound or free flow; reflects intense feelings, such as joy or anger, and an excitable temperament.

4. Low intensity

Tension remains moderately bound or free; reflects low-key reactions or decreased excitement, and a mild temperament.

5. Abrupt

Tension increases or decreases at a rapid rate; reflects impulsivity, impatience or alertness.

6. Gradual

Tension increases or decreases at a slow, leisurely rate; reflects patience, endurance, and taking the time to feel intensely. (Figure 2 is an example of the distribution of an individual's tension-flow attribute repertoire.)

Fetal Movement Notation

As already described, expectant parents begin their training in fetal movement notation with tension-flow touch attunement exercises. To illustrate this process further, in one exercise the expectant father presses his palms against the mother's back for a few seconds, then rhythmically releases

Figure 3. Fetal Movement Notation

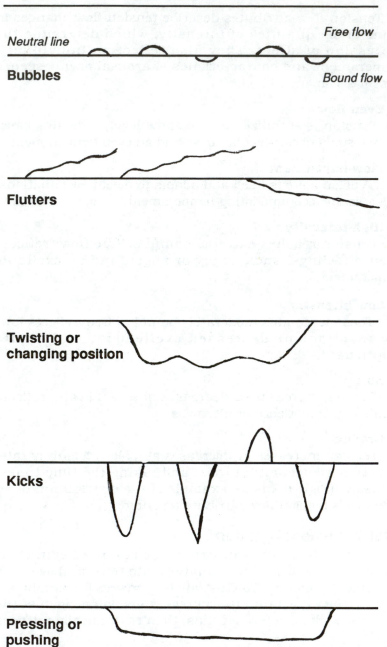

and repeats the pressure every few seconds. To attune with these sensations, the mother tenses and relaxes her fists in the same rhythm as the pressure. As she becomes adept at responding to these tension changes, she begins to isolate her responses to her hands and fingers.

The expectant mother traces the fetal movement notation on paper by hand. She can begin her fetal movement journal as early as the fourth or fifth month of pregnancy, and can either notate the movement as it occurs, or write it from memory. The notation records the variations in free and bound flow, rhythms and attributes along a time axis, which continues as long as the movement occurs. This time-line is the *Neutral Line*, dividing the area of free tension-flow above the line, from the area of bound tension-flow below the line. The further the perceived tension-flow is toward either extreme (free or bound), the further the corresponding notation will be from the Neutral Line. Therefore, high intensity free or bound flow is recorded far away from the Neutral Line, while low intensity flow is recorded near it. Gradual changes of tension-flow are indicated by gradually slanting lines, and abrupt changes are indicated by sharply slanting, peaked lines (Figure 3).

The process of kinesthetic attunement required for fetal movement notation creates the foundation for empathetic bonding between mother and unborn child. Other family members can also attune to the fetus by placing their hand on the expectant mother's abdomen, and simultaneously moving (pressing, twisting, adjusting, etc.) in response to fetal movement. In this way, they become acquainted with the new family member's movement preferences, and after birth, they feel a sense of familiarity with the new baby, because of their recognition of its unique movement patterns.

There is a great variety of fetal movement patterns. All the tension-flow rhythms, attributes, and combinations of rhythms and attributes can occur in the womb. Each individual fetus has its own unique movement repertoire. Furthermore, fetal movement appears to progress and develop over the course of the pregnancy. The early movements feel like small bubbles of low intensity and are fairly repetitive. As the pregnancy progresses, more variety of movement develops, and over time repeated movement phrases can be recognized. Some typical fetal movement patterns are shown in figure 3.

Some expectant mothers will feel a familiarity or compatibility with their unborn child's movement, while others will feel estranged from it. In either case, attunement to her fetus' movement can help the mother get to know her child and begin the process of mother-child bonding. On a family level, the individual tension-flow attribute diagrams of the fetus and other family members will show their characteristic patterns of temperament and affective expression. Therefore, these individual tension-flow diagrams can be used to improve understanding of potential areas of harmony and conflict within the family, and to assist the family system in adapting to the new addition.

Summary

The process of kinesthetic attunement, or empathetic identification, is necessary for notation of fetal movement. This attunement produces synchrony and mutual responsiveness to needs and feelings, as expressed through muscular tension-flow. It has also been shown to enhance communication and mutuality in families and relationships (Kestenberg, 1975; Sossin & Loman, 1982). Thus, early attunement with the fetus can provide the solid basis for empathetic understanding between parent and child. This fulfills one of the primary goals of the Prenatal Project, to prepare expectant parents not only for the birth process, but also for their relationship with the child.

Recommendations for Future Research

So far fetal movement notation has been used in a primary prevention setting with relatively high-functioning families. However, it may also be a powerful diagnostic tool. Since it requires complete empathetic attunement, parents who have difficulty with fetal movement notation may be prime candidates for additional training in parenting skills. Therefore, it could be used in a secondary prevention setting, to identify expectant mothers who have difficulty relating nonverbally to their fetus. Interventions could then be initiated to provide these mothers with extra support and training.

Another application of fetal attunement might be with adoptive families, before or after the adoption, or in a clinical setting. Adoptive parents do not have the opportunity to familiarize themselves with their new child through fetal movement notation. To overcome this deficit, touch attunement exercises could be taught to adoptive parents to teach them to recognize and respond to their children's needs and to enhance early communication.

Follow-up research with families in the fetal movement notation classes could study their relationship with the child over time. This research would observe the long-term effects of the training, and could be compared to a control group to discover any differences with families who have not been trained.

Finally, more professionals working with expectant families should be trained in the KMP, in order to expand the study and application of fetal movement notation in research, prevention and therapy.

References

Amoruso, L. (1982). A special thank you. Child Development Research News, 5 (1).

Bartenieff, I. & Lewis, D. (1980). Body movement: Coping with the environment. New York: Gordon and Breach.

Chace, M. (1975). Dance as an adjunctive therapy with hospitalized mental patients. In H. Chaikin, (Ed.), Marian Chace: Her papers. Columbia, MD: American Dance Therapy Association.

Freud, A. (1965). Normality and pathology in childhood: Assessments of development. In The writings of Anna Freud (Vol. 6). New York: International Universities Press.

Jordan, S. (1981). The prenatal program. Child Development

Research News, 3 (2).

Kestenberg, J. S. (1975). Children and parents: Psychoanalytic studies in development. New York: Jason Aronson.

Kestenberg, J. S. (1976). Regression and reintegration in pregnancy. Journal of the American Psychoanalytic Association, 24, 213-250.

Kestenberg, J. S. (1980). Pregnancy as a developmental phase. Journal of Biological Experience: Studies in the Life of the Body, 3, 58.

Kestenberg, J. S. (1982). Parenthood — A changing lifestyle. Child Development Research News, 4 (2).

Kestenberg, J. S. (1985). The role of movement patterns in diagnosis and prevention. In D.A. Shoskan & W.L. Roller (Eds.), Paul Schilder: Mind explorer. New York: Human Sciences Press, Inc.

Kestenberg, J. S., Marcus, H., Robbins, E., Berlow, J., & Buelte, A. (1975). Children and parents: Psychoanalytic studies in development. New York: Jason Aronson.

Kestenberg, J. S. & Sossin, M. (1979). The role of movement patterns in development (Vol. 2). New York: Dance Notation Bureau Press.

Lamb, W. (1965). Posture and Gesture. London: Gerald Duckworth.

Loman, S. (1980). The Prenatal Project. Child Development Research News, 2 (1).

Loman, S., Aigen, K., & Leevwenburgh, E. (1988, October). Non-verbal empathy with infants and toddlers through movement, music and art. Paper presented at the Kids in Crisis Conference sponsored by the Center for Creative Art Therapies, Cambridge, MA.

Sossin, K. & Loman, S. (1982, October). Clinical applications of the Kestenberg Movement Profile: Diagnosis and treatment. Paper presented at the American Dance Therapy Association Annual Conference, Rye, NY.

Notes

[1] I have participated in the Preparation for the Child classes, and used fetal movement notation during pregnancy with both of my children. Some of my personal experiences and observations may therefore be of interest to the reader. Fetal movement notation gave me a vivid sense of pre-natal bonding and post-natal recognition with both of my sons, who have very different innate personalities. Their fetal movements were also very different, enabling me to become familiar with their dominant personality traits in utero (which have continued in their subsequent development). During my first pregnancy, I played folk music and Mozart through earphones to my son. He would respond either with no movement (sleeping?) or with rhythmic activity. The same music appeared to soothe him after birth. He now appears to be very musical, and especially loves Mozart. Incidentally, his strongest movement response in utero was to a high note sung by a tenor at an opera performance — it is possible that he was agitated by its volume and high frequency.

Movement Retraining

Arnhilt Buelte

Introduction

Movement observation, notation and interpretation are critical means of studying early development and are used at the Center for Parents and Children as the basis for movement intervention, which we[1] call Movement Retraining. Retraining is done with children and parents individually and in groups. Some of the goals are: to help parents attune to their children's changing and maturing movement patterns in all of the developmental phases; to help children achieve mastery of the developmental tasks of each phase; and to teach parents to provide the structure necessary for the achievement of mastery in each specific phase. This involves helping parents develop supportive interventions which stimulate and encourage the practice of phase-appropriate movement patterns.

This paper summarizes the normal sequence of movement patterns necessary for coping with the physical environment from infancy through the walking-running stage. It includes examples of specific Movement Retraining interventions to help young children practice and master each phase. Since specific forms of holding or supporting are necessary at each stage, this paper also emphasizes the importance of proper holding and supporting by parents to enable the child to control emerging movement patterns. Through this support and attunement, parents provide the necesssary structure for the child to go through each developmental phase with a feeling of success rather than failure.

Editor's Note: The feminine gender is used to refer to the baby or child throughout this article both for clarity and ease of reading and to offer some balance to the predominant use of the masculine gender in most publications.

Movement work with parents is another vital aspect of Movement Retraining. Retraining classes include exercises which help parents to re-experience movement patterns that are abundant in infants and toddlers. Being able to re-experience in their own bodies what young children feel and finding ways of coping with the physical environment through movement will help parents better attune to their children's needs and provide a supportive structure for their developmental progression.

In the first and second years of life, changes in a child's movement repertoire appear almost daily at first, and then almost weekly. By recognizing gross and subtle changes, we can pinpoint the height of each developmental stage, as well as the especially sensitive transitions between phases and between sub-phases. We are becoming more and more aware of the vulnerability of these transitional periods.

Each of the developmental phases requires its own form of holding and support-giving. The phases described here are nursing, sitting, crawling, standing, walking sideways, walking, and preparation for climbing.

Nursing

An early example of movement attunement can be seen during nursing. The feeling of well-being between mother and infant, and the success of breast-feeding depend on the mother cradling the infant by supporting her head, back and legs (which should be in contact with her mother's torso, not hanging from the mother's arm or knees). Supported in this way, the appropriate breathing pattern of **widening** into her mother's arm and towards her body, followed by **narrowing** back, can occur. Success depends, furthermore, on the child being held firmly (but not in high intensity) with enough space that her hands and body can move in the rhythm of nursing. Lastly, success depends on the mother's ability to respond to her movements in the same or a similar rhythm. Retraining helps mother and child to achieve the delicate balance of bodily comfort and attunement.

Sitting

When a baby is first placed in a sitting position, she will slump forward, often with a bobbing head, or shrink into her body, as if lacking a neck. We show parents how to support the baby by holding a hand against her back, and how to adjust their own bodies so that she feels a firm support when leaning against them. Supported like this, the baby's spine lengthens and one can feel and see how the lengthening continues into her head. She then learns to control this movement autonomously, first by holding up her head and later by sitting erect.

Crawling

A sitting child has learned to support the upper part of her torso, while the lower part is still supported by the chair, lap or floor. When a toy is put in front of her, just out of reach, she will lean her upper torso forward and reach out to get it. If she leans too far forward, she may lose her balance, landing face down on her chest and stomach with legs on the side in a frog-like position. In order to move forward from this position beyond her reach, the child must learn to coordinate upper and lower parts of her body, pulling her legs underneath her body and pushing her chest away from the floor. This requires control over **high-intensity, low-intensity** and **twisting**[2] movement patterns, which will eventually enable the child to crawl. This is a major achievement on the road to adaptation to the physical forces of the environment; for the first time, she is able to move away from or toward a person or object on her own — the first form of locomotion. Until now, everything was brought to her, or she was carried from place to place.

In this phase, mothers often experience an ambivalent feeling: pride over their children's achievement and sadness over their moving away in space — a first form of separation. However, a crawling child will sit down often, turning her body sideways to face the direction she came from. With a smile of relief, she will recognize her mother, expecting her to be where she left her, and then go back to exploring the environment.

The crawling child is a true explorer of the surrounding space. This is sometimes difficult for parents since everything in the now very-mobile child's reach will be touched and investigated. Well-meaning parents, trying to protect the child, often curtail the crawler's activities by pulling her away from dangerous situations and sitting her on the floor or on someone's lap. The child's body receives the message not to crawl. We encourage parents to "child-proof" their homes rather than to discourage the urge to crawl, which is a crucial step towards exploration of the environment.

We try to help children achieve mastery over the developmental task of crawling by, at the right time, stimulating and integrating their control over the increasingly more complex movement patterns. In crawling, children learn to diagonally connect the upper and lower parts of the body. Lifting the abdomen away from the floor strengthens the abdominal muscles, and shifting the weight from one side to the other helps to develop automatic control over the center of gravity — a prerequisite for standing.

Standing

Having integrated and mastered the movement patterns of crawling, children become very interested in vertical obstacles, like a bookshelf, a couch or a low table. They will look up, reach up and kneel in front of these objects. We can facilitate success with the next stage by providing a stable object at shoulder height that they can reach from a kneeling position. The culminating moment comes when, holding on to this object, they place one foot flat on the floor and then simultaneously push down and lengthen up from the inner center of the body, the center of gravity, to reach a standing position.

What an accomplishment this is! The whole body becomes one solid piece, with upper and lower parts connected, the boundaries sharply defined, and the knees locked. However, holding this one-piece posture makes it difficult to lower the body to the floor again. Some children just give in to gravity and plop down, while others become frustrated, holding themselves in **high-intensity**, making it even harder to go down. Children slowly learn, sometimes with our help, to lower their intensity of vertical holding and to allow the integration of gradual tension changes into their movements. This will enable them to practice and eventually master the task of standing, stooping and standing up again to confront the world and their parents as autonomous individuals.

Moving Sideways

The standing child's pride in mastering the force of gravity is so contagious that parents and observers usually react with a feeling of pride and relief. Finally, the days of crawling on the floor seem to be over, and the child is expected to move around on two feet like the rest of us. Adults stretch out their hands, motioning or saying "come here." However, a child who has just learned to stand is firmly aligned in the vertical plane — she feels the boundaries of her body as having width and height. She protects these boundaries by holding herself firmly in a one-piece posture, often in high intensity, in order not to lose her emerging control over gravity.

Her movement out of this alignment is not going forward but taking steps sideways, holding on to an object (first for support and later for guidance). A child will move sideways along coffee tables, chairs and low wall shelves, occasionally letting go for a moment to reach sideways for the next object. Providing opportunities for these sideways movements allows children to learn, and later master, control over **high-** and **low-intensity** changes from the center of gravity, a pre-requisite for using **strength** and **lightness** in walking and climbing. Therefore, children should be given ample opportunity to develop this sense of balance. If a child does require support at this time, we recommend putting both hands lightly around her waist for stabilization. If she is held by her outstretched arms, as is often done, her shoulders will lock in high intensity, and her waist will become wobbly. This conflicts with her emerging postural stability necessary for good self-representation.

When a child at this stage has the urge to move somewhere quickly, she will get down on her hands and knees and rapidly crawl to her destination, using the most efficient form of locomotion. This is perfectly phase-appropriate; she is still integrating her newly-developed control over **high-** and **low-intensity** and beginning **strength** and **lightness** with the previously accomplished control over **even** and **fluctuating flow** and beginning **directness** and **indirectness**. Having reached the object of her interest, she will stand up again, holding on and eventually letting go of the support. She will stoop down more and more, stay in a stooped position longer, pick up objects and stand up holding them. Children at this stage like to climb over small hurdles and into and out of boxes, tires and other obstacles. Again, if help is needed, only light support around the waist is recommended.

The satisfaction of conquering the force of gravity to face and confront the larger world is so great, that children will practice until they have fully mastered the task. To allow a child to gain mastery with a feeling of achievement rather than failure, it is essential for adults to recognize the difference between support and the fostering of premature movement patterns. A standing child, as she practices moving sideways alongside furniture in a wide stance with great stability, is still aligned in the vertical plane. At this point, she often stands up holding on to her parent's leg. The adult is tempted to slowly walk forward, hoping the child will walk along with him. If a child tries this, her arms tense around her parent's leg, her torso bends forward at the waist, and she soon loses vertical balance and falls. A beginning walker does not need a physical stimulus to move forward. These stimuli only send her the message that she is not able to walk by herself.

Walking Forward

When children have developed a good sense of balance and are able to step sideways, using objects only for guidance, not support, they are ready to finally move forward. Where they would previously have gone down on their knees to crawl to their destination, now they stand in a body attitude of acute preparedness to walk. However, breaking out of vertical alignment and just-mastered vertical balance is difficult. Responding to the increasing natural influx of small gradual and **abrupt** tension-flow changes, and to the increasing urge to move into the sagittal plane, will impel them to take those first steps at the right time — in a wide stance, one foot forward, and then the other. This gets them out of the vertical alignment into a forward motion. An object or person is often the initial aim, but the first steps also show the child's entrancement with simply moving forward autonomously in space. If over-excitement leads to a fall, children will sit or stand up by themselves. Getting up by oneself is an achievement; being picked up and carried away is not! Proper support in this situation simply reuqires being present to watch a child cope with his emerging control over new movement elements.

A beginning walker often leans her torso forward, only the balls of her feet touching the floor, which can lead to a fall. At this point, adults usually offer their hands as support. Most likely, the child will have to tense her shoulders to counteract the pull from above, obscuring the subtle changes in her torso, legs and hips needed for the new kind of balance, making her prone to falling. Given time to practice on her own, (with only slight support at the waist, if necessary), she will learn to put her weight on the whole foot, to bring both feet closer together, and to bend her knees in harmony with her leg's rotation in the hipjoint.

Through control over **gradual** and **abrupt** tension changes and integration with previously mastered movement patterns, children balance themselves in the sagittal plane — forward and backward. Their arms, outstretched like airplane wings, help them balance at first, and then begin to swing in rhythm with their gait. Children practice walking and running — falling at first — until they can stop at will and break the fall. Toddlers are preoccupied with walking and running, and their delight in their new-found mobility is contagious, if at times hard for their parents to cope with.

At this point, parents often hold the child's hand in public, for safety reasons. Since it is uncomfortable for the adult to bend down to provide a balancing support, we often see children almost hanging on an adult's arm with no possibility of supporting themselves and controlling their own movements. Awareness of this problem can motivate parents to find other ways of walking at their child's pace and holding hands at the child's level without pulling.

Preparation for Climbing

Stepping up and down prefigures the maturation of climbing skills. One can already observe a form of pre-climbing in a young baby when she is held so that infant and adult can breathe in attunement. Facing the adult, firmly supported under the buttocks in a pre-sitting position with the upper torso resting on the adult's chest, the baby will pull her legs under her body and crawl up the chest. This response to optimal holding and support is first a reflex but soon becomes a controlled movement. Crawling up the parent's chest gives the child an early sensation of moving upward, which is similiar to climbing. However, the infant is still completely dependent on being held and supported in this first climbing experience.

When a child starts to crawl, she will often move toward a person who is sitting on the floor. She will try to climb over the adult's legs and up his torso. Parents can provide support by sitting so that the child will not fall over their legs, and lose her balance, experiencing failure. When the child crawls upward onto their bodies (pulling up, rather than standing up), adults can place both hands around her waist, gently but firmly, to help her experience the connection between her upper and lower body.

Next, a young crawler will head toward other objects, such as steps, which she will climb up with great enjoyment. To be successful, she must learn to control **high-** and **low-intensity** from her center of gravity, and to coordinate this with her already-achieved control over **even** and **fluctuating flow** changes. This, in turn, will help her master more mature movement patterns, which will enable her to stand up instead of pull up into a standing position.

After watching a child climb up a flight of stairs, parents will often pick the child up and carry her down. This action leads her to expect that parents will be there at all times. An important support in this phase is helping her crawl down the steps backwards on her belly on her own. This requires time and patience. At first, the child has to be turned onto her belly and helped down by having her feet placed on each step against an initial intense resistance (the urge is to go up instead of down). However, she soon learns and enjoys being able to move down backwards speedily and independently. This prepares her for the more difficult task of going up and down stairs, and later climbing jungle gyms and other playground equipment.

Going up and down stairs successfully is a true test of the integration of old and newly-mastered movement elements, requiring the coordination of many complex factors. In walking up, these factors are: **direct** placement of the foot with flow changes and **indirectness** in the hip and knee, use of **strength** and **lightness** from the center of the body (changing the weight in relation to gravity), **acceleration** to move the body into the sagittal plane, and **deceleration** to change feet. This is a tremendous task, which requires support from hands or a railing at first. Stepping down is even more difficult. The same movement elements must be integrated in a different order.

Let us look at an example of stepping down just one step. When an early walker approaches a curb, usually a helping hand is offered. Stepping down, the child will often almost hang on the adult's hand without any feeling of self-support. Given the opportunity to approach a curb at her own pace, a child will hesitate in preparation, look down, realize the difference in height (more so than going up), and recognize the challenge she is facing. At this point a supportive hand is helpful, but just for balance — not for leading! The child, when ready, will step down — and be so elated about this achievement that she will most likely turn around to practice again and again. Success at stepping down triggers a stimulus in the child's body which prepares her for one aspect of future jumping which will be learned, practiced, and mastered in a later phase.

Summary

The sequential emergence and maturation of movement patterns extends through adulthood; this paper deals with Retraining from infancy to the walking stage. In the Retraining of infants and young children, we aim to foster optimal development in the first years of life. We place special emphasis on noticing the emergence of phase-appropriate movement elements, encouraging the practice of these patterns and recognizing the mastery of the developmental task in each phase. Early intervention in all phases, especially in transitional phases, where children are most vulnerable, will prevent difficulties in later life. In Movement Retraining of adults, we teach parents the different forms of support, holding, attunement and structuring, required in each developmental phase. Movement Retraining assists children and parents in successfully meeting the challenges in each period of early development.

_____

Notes

[1]The author was Co-Director of the Center for Parents and Children in Roslyn, New York from 1972 to 1990. This paper describes her work at the Center, and is based on a series of articles which first appeared in Child Development Research News (1:1, 1:2, 2:1, 2:2, 4:2, 5:1, 6:1, 6:2) from 1978 to 1984.

[2]For definitions of movement terms (in boldface), the reader is referred to Kestenberg & Sossin (1979). The role of movement patterns in development: Vol. 2. New York: Dance Notation Bureau Press.

Part II:
Expanding and Bridging
the KMP Perspective

Nonverbal Communication of Affect in Bali: Movement in Parenting and Dance

Janet Kestenberg-Amighi, Ph.D.
Islene Pinder
Judith S. Kestenberg, M.D.

Introduction

Philosophers like to ask their students whether a tree in the lifeless desert makes any sound when it falls. In other words, if there are no ears to hear, does a falling tree make a sound? While philosophers may ponder, social scientists have no problem with this question. They would say that it all depends on how you define "sound." Unfortunately, relying on operational definitions, as social scientists and psychologists do, is not as good a solution as it might be. Some psychologists, for example, have defined maternal affect as the number of times a mother looks at her child, kisses it, and coos to it, in five ten-minute samplings. While we question this as a valid measure of affect in our culture, it is even more questionable when applied *a priori* to other cultures.

At the other extreme, Margaret Mead suggested that to understand another culture, we must completely drop all of our preconceived notions of how reality is structured. Looking at what appears to be a house, we must allow ourselves only to see pieces of wood held together by nails. We must be reborn again, as children looking about us and seeing things for the first time (Mead, 1972). Although this idea sounds good, most anthropologists today would say that it is an unrealistic goal. We can never dismantle our culturally structured view of the world. Even as anthropologists, we are fated to see only our own version of reality (Marcus & Fischer, 1986). As with most important controversies, it seems that there is an ingredient of truth in both views. Preconceived categories distort, and reality without categories is unknowable.

A partial integration of these two positions may be gained by combining the traditional participation-observation approach of anthropology (geared to learning native categories) with a more formal and systematic method of data collection, which does not impose Western cultural categories on its subjects. As suggested elsewhere (Kestenberg-Amighi,1990), the Kestenberg Movement Profile (KMP) may be such a methodology. That it relies on elemental forms of movement, rather than on culturally defined modes of affect expression, has been supported by comparisons of clinical data from the United States and Israel. The KMP exhibits a reasonable degree of inter-observer reliability among trained notators. Furthermore, KMP data can be gathered on children in their normal settings, without the disruption of laboratory tests. We hope that comparison of our field data, and that of other anthropologists, such as Bateson and Mead (1942), Geertz (1973) and Wikan (1989), will support its validity in cross-cultural settings.

This paper presents the preliminary findings of our study of Balinese infants and adults. Only a small number of the profiles have been analyzed to date, and thus our interpretations are still subject to reformulation. The fieldwork for this study was undertaken by Islene Pinder and Janet Kestenberg-Amighi, and the profiles were constructed and interpreted by Judith Kestenberg, M.D.

This paper is divided into three sections. We will begin by discussing the controversy in the literature concerning affect expression and the need for better measures of affect. This controversy extends into the case of Bali, and its specifics will be outlined for the reader. Secondly, we will suggest that movement analysis in the study of affect is particularly appropriate in cultures such as Bali, where kinesthetic modes of communication are predominant. We will also consider the general context of Balinese culture in understanding affect expression. Finally, we will review the results of six profiles and consider how these results integrate with the descriptive material of the literature on Bali. Since this is a work in progress, our results are preliminary.

Operational Definition of Affect Communication

Cultures may possibly be classified into two categories: those in which distal modes of affect communication, i.e., verbal/auditory and visual, are dominant and those in which near modes of communication, primarily kinesthetic, are dominant (Brazelton, 1977; Goldberg, 1977). Of course, all modes are used in all cultures, so these differences are a matter of emphasis. In tropical climates we generally find a high degree of body contact between infant and mother (and other caretakers), throughout the early years. LeVine and LeVine have suggested that this serves to protect infants from environmental hazards in cultures where high infant mortality creates a focus on their physical survival (1981).

In addition to a high level of body contact, many investigators have reported a low level of eye-to-eye contact, smiling and verbalization between mother and infant among tropical agriculturists (Ainsworth, 1967; Dixon, et al, 1981). It has been suggested that this indicates a lower degree of affective communication than in Western cultures (LeVine, 1977; Dixon, et al, 1981). The question arises, however, whether there is not affective and cognitive communication between parents and infant in the kinesthetic mode, which has escaped the attention of earlier investigators. In other words, is it not ethnocentric to focus on distal modes of communication and other popularly defined measures of affect? In a cross-cultural study of maternal affect, Lewis and Ban used the usual "how many times per time sampling period the mother engaged in behaviors such as looking, touching, smiling, playing, vocalizing." But they also questioned whether more cross-cultural similarities would not be found if more "proper" variables were used (1977).

Thus, we turn to a combination of naturalistic observations and the KMP to enable us to discover and measure the elusive components of affect communication.

Affect Communication in Bali

The Balinese culture is particularly interesting for the study of nonverbal affect communication. According to their cultural rules, strong emotions such as fear, anger, and love are to be expressed only in a subdued manner, or not at all. It is considered proper to present oneself to the world as a smooth, unruffled individual (see Wikan, 1989). Men and women are not to publicly show affection to each other. Any aggressive display of emotions is not accepted and is frightening to others. An individual who appears to be emotionally out of control is considered to be under the influence of black magic.

Geertz has suggested that the Balinese engage in a "thorough-going attempt to block individuality, spontaneity and emotionality . . . from sight . . . through formality, ceremony, and convention." (Geertz, 1973, p. 388). Another anthropologist, Unni Wikan, focuses on day-to-day life rather than rules and ideals. She points out that Balinese people have turbulent hearts; they do cry and lose their tempers, but she agrees that it does not happen often. They are continually engaged in what she calls "emotion work." They offer the viewer a cheerful face and bright smile, "in an effort to 'not care'" (1987 , p. 339). They use this surface persona to protect the self against experiencing or showing intense feelings.

The Balinese live with a powerful paradox. On one hand, they see their lives as inextricably bound with others. They are parts of families and groups and declare themselves happy only when with other people. On the other hand, they are continually afraid that friends as well as strangers may be offended by them and strike them with black magic. Pinder has never met a Balinese who did not have concerns about black magic. There are numerous stories of individuals who were entered by demonic forces because their neighbor was jealous and made a contract with a balian or witch doctor. Thus, a Balinese must always walk cautiously; both taking in the support of others, and yet guarding against their possible malevolence (Wikan, 1989). Thus, they must always exhibit a bright and cheerful face.

Although Geertz focuses on the symbolic world and the aesthetic, and Wikan focuses on the experiential world and the fear of witchcraft, they both see the end result as a severely curtailed expression of affect. Feelings, though sometimes strong, are carefully hidden.

A visitor to Bali would probably quickly agree with the

portrait drawn by Geertz and Wikan. Balinese walk down the road with empty, neutral faces. They greet a visitor with a careful smile, and little of the profusion of pleasure found in middle eastern and many western cultures. The Balinese are routinely friendly and helpful, but restrained. It is difficult to discover whether your visit is appreciated or not. But are these outsider's observations a good measure of interpersonal affect communication within the community?

According to several Balinese friends and acquaintances, the Balinese are emotional people who speak from the liver (heart), in contrast to the rather cold foreigners, who may use good words but do not speak from the heart. This seems to indicate that the nonverbal or kinesthetic mode of communication is where we should look for affect communication, and that its form might be on a more basic level than facial expression or gesture.

The Kinesthetic Mode of Affect Communication

Islene Pinder first visited Bali in 1976, to study dance with a famous teacher. In the course of her dance studies, she became intrigued with Balinese child rearing practices. As she studied both areas simultaneously, she was struck by a shared feature: for training dancers and raising infants, the Balinese use a process we have termed kinesthetic shaping. Pinder began to see the kinesthetic sphere as integral to understanding both Balinese dance and Balinese child rearing, and she sought out a methodology for data collection and analysis of the kinesthetic sphere. To our great fortune, she turned to the study of the KMP. So began our collaboration, with Islene Pinder as film-maker and student of Balinese culture, Janet Kestenberg-Amighi as anthropologist and KMP profiler, and Mark Sossin and Judith Kestenberg as consulting experts in the KMP.

Further study of Pinder's videotapes convinced us that the kinesthetic sphere was indeed critical to many aspects of Balinese life. We used three approaches to understanding Balinese culture through the kinesthetic sphere: the KMP, interviewing, and participation observation. We hoped that the validity of the KMP data would be supported or refuted by our use of two supplementary data collection methodologies, as well as by comparisons with the literature.

Our thesis that kinesthetic empathy and interaction is the primary mode of affect communication in Balinese culture. Below we describe the use of the kinesthetic mode in several different settings.

Balinese child rearing involves a considerable amount of tactile stimulation and holding. Babies are bathed and massaged twice a day. The belief is that the face and body can be made more beautiful through massage. In addition, mothers hold their children or lie next to them during nursing, sleep with them, and carry them about for much of the day. Mothers will also give their child to the father or siblings for care. This means that premobile infants spend few waking hours that are not in physical contact with another human being.

While massaging or bathing the baby, mothers often engage in conversation with relatives or co-wives lingering about the courtyard. Socially engaged with others, they do not make frequent eye contact with the infant, nor usually sing or talk to them. However, throughout nursing and bathing, they hold, touch and manipulate the infant. This focus on the kinesthetic not only reinforces its importance as a channel for communication and learning, but also singles it out as distinct from others. It may also diminish the importance of other channels (i.e., verbal ones).

Kinesthetic communication also forms an integral part of Balinese dance training. While most Western dancers learn by using auditory, visual, and kinesthetic modes, Balinese children appear to be taught to focus primarily on the kinesthetic mode, through external kinesthetic shaping as well as internal kinesthetic feedback. In external kinesthetic shaping, the instructor holds the student from behind, dancing with them and moving their arms, body and legs in the expected shapes and rhythms of the dance. Both male and female instructors commonly use **bound flow**, aggressive movements and intrusive rhythms, such as slashes, punches and presses. Students appear to accept the intrusions without resistance.

Even while watching the dance instructor, the student's focus is on incorporating the right feeling tones through kinesthetic attunement with the instructor. Sometimes students dance without watching anyone, focusing inward, using only the rhythm of the gamelan orchestra.

The dance postures of both female and male dancers are unusual and initially uncomfortable positions into which the body is forced. They are quite different than the natural everyday posture of Balinese men and women. The message appears to be that outer forces direct and shape the behavior of the individual. These outer influences are incorporated and internalized in dance, just as in child rearing.

In some parts of Bali, dancers fall into trance. They explain that they are invaded by spirits, ancestral or other. Friends and kinsmen hold the person to keep them from doing damage to themselves, and lead them in a procession out of the temple and into the streets. These trance dancers will take a sword and press it to their chest, but will not be hurt because the spirits are protecting them. This is another example of taking in outside influences and incorporating them, allowing them to control one's movements, even one's hand on a sword.

The kinesthetic mode of affect communication is often used in preference to the verbal one. Balinese friends are often in physical contact while joking and laughing together. A Balinese may offer what we would consider a minimal greeting, and then settle easily beside the visitor, leaning or resting an arm on them.

There also appears to be a form of noncontact kinesthetic attunement. In both family and non-family groups, one can observe Balinese shift their positions in unison. Even without physical contact, attunement takes place. In everyday life, Balinese are involved in enormous and serious responsibilities to their temples, gods, village, family, ancestors, and guilds (Geertz & Geertz, 1975). Elaborate towers, sculptures, and offerings are constructed by groups of people on a regular basis. The timing and rhythm of the groups' activities are measured and exact. Geertz has called it a choreographed mob scene (1980). Yet a director is often absent.

The space between people is socially significant. The Balinese say that they like a crowded or populated environment (ramai) and are depressed by empty space (spi). They may have no noticable interaction with any other person in the space, but the presence of others affects them emotionally.

Space populated by other people is comforting and meaningful. This is particularly noticeable at funerals, where the chief mourners are not surrounded by others offering murmurs of sympathy, hugs or hand holds. They often stand alone or wander amongst the crowds of people in neutral flow. From the Western viewpoint, they appear neglected. But the Balinese insist, "No, they are not alone. We are here for them, and do not let them be alone for one minute for the first seventy hours."

The Balinese express deep feelings through subtle, modulated gestures and bodily movements. A few of these movements have been recognized by Western observers. Bateson and Mead described the "look away" detached stance (1942). When a woman broke into tears over an insult from a relative, her husband withdrew from her, looking away. He removed himself from her unacceptable emotional behavior, clearly conveying his disapproval without words. The withdrawal, the sulk, the lookaway, the slow walk, are subtle but describable expressions of affect. However, it is likely that other movements which communicate affect to Balinese are unobserved or misunderstood by members of a foreign culture.

The difficulty arises not only from the barriers to cross-cultural understanding, but also because of the complexity of Balinese emotional expression. The Balinese attempt to subdue their own emotions and emotional expression, and at the same time, seek to understand the emotions of others. They try to be empathetic with others, while maintaining a cautious barrier between themselves and others. This apparent conflict points towards the importance of exploring nonverbal forms of affect expression.

Findings of the KMP

The main focus of the preliminary analysis is on discovering movement patterns common to all 24 individuals studied, in dance, child rearing, and everyday activities, patterns which might be characteristic of the culture. Videos of movements were made by Islene Pinder and Janet Kestenberg-Amighi and the profiles were developed by Judith Kestenberg. We were ultimately interested in discovering modes of affect expression and communication from the KMP analysis.

1. We found a characteristic sequence of rhythms of

tension-flow used by all participants in the study: six mothers, six fathers, six babies, and three male and three female Balinese dancers. This sequence is composed primarily of **oral aggressive** (biting) rhythms and **outer genital** (intrusive) rhythms. The mixture of outer genital libidinal and oral aggressive is a movement which intrudes, clings fleetingly, not wanting to let go, but then withdraws abruptly. In our videos, we frequently see older children darting into the space of a toddler, poking, prodding, and then withdrawing as quickly as they came. Mothers also use such patterns in the way they feed toddlers who are on the run.

Toddlers usually respond to the frequent intrusions by going into a **neutral flow** — passively accepting. Picked up and twirled around, or being moved in step to a dance rhythm, toddlers often become deanimated like dolls, their eyes glazing over. They use this neutral flow as a primary defense against intrusions. This does not mean that they do not sometimes enjoy the attention that they are receiving. Remember that the intrusions are done with indulging rhythms. The neutral flow response means that they are conditioned to respond to high levels of stimulation with diminished responses, whether the stimulation is pleasant or unpleasant. This is reminiscent of Bateson and Mead's report that when Balinese are under a high degree of stress, they often go to sleep (1942). However, a trancelike state is also reached in response to pleasant stimuli, such as when an infant is massaged in its twice daily bath.

Thus, from infancy through adulthood, we see two common patterns of interaction: the intrusive, briefly clinging or persisting approach and the response of neutral flow deanimation. Neutral flow may be interpreted by the outside observer as a negation of affect communication, but it may actually signal acceptance to the Balinese.

2. Overall indulging rhythms are more prevalent than fighting rhythms. This indicates that the Balinese studied have more drives directed towards pleasure-seeking than fighting. A high oral score can be related

to the Balinese emphasis on taking in outside influences, a focus of early childhood training.

3. The rhythms are often mixed and/or undifferentiated among the adults, at a level higher than is usually found among American adults. The two interesting exceptions to this pattern were the newborn infants who had more clearly differentiated drive patterns than the adults. This was a surprising result. If confirmed, it indicates that Balinese infants are born with a high degree of drive organization, but gradually diminish their capacity to differentiate one drive wish from another, as they are taught to submerge their needs to the needs of the family and the community as a whole.

4. We found that in all individuals there were more tension-flow attributes than tension-flow rhythms, which indicates more emphasis on feelings than on needs. Furthermore, the tension flow attributes (affects) have a high degree of complexity. The presence of well-differentiated and well-integrated emotions would seem to contradict Geertz's description of the Balinese as a people with low affects and confirm the Balinese view of themselves as highly emotional people (Wikan, 1989). But what happens to these emotions? Why do their affects appear to be so minimal to outside observers? We can look for the answer in their patterns of free, bound and neutral flow and in their patterns of bipolar shape flow:

a. We found a widespread prevalence of **bound flow** over **free flow**, indicating that these complex emotions are often expresed with caution. We also found a consistently high level of **neutral flow**, which deadens the expression of emotion. It would be important to discover under what circumstances bound flow or neutral flow is used.

b. We can also consider their bipolar shape flow patterns, which most clearly reveal feelings to outsiders, as they provide the structure for emotional expression. In Balinese bipolar shape flow, we find a high ratio of bipolar **growing movements** (which generally express feelings of comfort, happiness and self confidence) to **shrinking** movements (which express discomfort, unhappiness, and lack of self-confidence). This means that Balinese express their feelings of happiness more than they express their feelings of unhappiness. This clearly fits into the cultural rules. However, it is interesting that even when expressing the culturally acceptable happiness, affects are expressed with more **bound flow** (caution) than **free flow**. In movement terms, we can say that in the majority of Balinese studied, the bipolar shape-flow and the tension-flow diagrams are not well matched, since they tend to use bound flow to accompany growing movements.

When bipolar movements, by which we generally intuit the mood and feelings of another person, are mismatched with tension flow, the dynamics of these feelings, interpretation of affect becomes very difficult. Feelings must be understood less through shape-flow and more through tension-flow, less through visual stimuli and more through kinesthetic attunement.

5. Looking at pre-efforts (defenses) and efforts (ways of adapting to reality), we find that the latter are more pronounced. This can be interpreted to mean that more energy is devoted to coping with reality, meeting every day survival tasks, than dealing with inner conflicts. The basic defenses of **bound flow** and **neutral flow** are relied upon, rather than the more complex pre-efforts.

6. Finally, we note that among mothers and fathers and among male and female dancers an interesting inversion takes place. Males tend to use more **inner genital** flowing rhythms, while females use more **outer genital** or jumping rhythms. This is interesting, given that in Ubud Bali, where our data was collected, many of the men are artists or dancers who work at home, while their wives often work in small shops. Therefore, the men sometimes spend long hours with their children, although grandmothers and siblings also play an active role. We may ask whether child care promotes indulgent inner genital rhythms among men, a pattern which may be initiated when young boys are pressed

into child care service, or whether there are other important factors, such as the form of parenting of boys versus girls. Further investigation will be required before attempting to address this issue.

Conclusions

How well does the above analysis reflect or shed light on Balinese culture as interpreted by traditional antropologists? The results given here are abbreviated and preliminary, based as they are on a very small sample. As we collect more data on our sample of six children each year, we will gain more knowledge of developmental patterns, training in the Balinese forms of emotional expression, and other areas, from observation and profile analysis.

At this point, we are nonetheless pleased to see that the preliminary results concur with inferences made by ourselves and other anthropologists on the basis of traditional observations. Our data tends to support the interpretation of Wikan over Geertz (although we note that Geertz deals with the symbolic rather than behavioral domain). More specifically, the presence of complex affect expressed with caution (**bound flow**), supports Wikan's portrayal of the Balinese as people who work hard to contain their "turbulent" emotions. The high use of neutral flow, however, indicates that deadening of emotions is also a feature of the Balinese cultural repertoire. More attention to the context of these two flow patterns is now required. In other words, under what circumstances are emotions carefully controlled and under what circumstances are they numbed? It is important to remember that complex affects can coexist with a numbed deanimated look. Finally, we are intrigued by the inverted movement patterns of males and females. We seek to discover how these relate to maternal/paternal roles and gender-related child-raising patterns in Balinese culture.

References

Ainsworth, M. (1967). Infancy in Uganda: Infant care and the growth of love. Baltimore: John Hopkins Press.

Bateson, G. & Mead, M. (1942). Balinese Character: A Photographic Analysis. Special Publication. New York Academy of Science, vol. 2. New York.

Brazelton, T. (1977). Implications of infant development among the Mayan Indians of Mexico. In P. Eiderman, S. Tullein & A. Rosenfield (Eds.), Culture and infancy (pp. 151-188). New York: Academic Press.

Dixon, S., Tronick, E., Keefer, C., & Brazelton, T. (1981). Mother-infant interaction among the Gusii of Kenya. In T. Field, A. Sostek, P. Vietze & P. Liederman (Eds.), Culture and early interaction. Hillsdale, New Jersey: Lawrence Erlbaum Associates.

Geertz, C. (1973). Person, time, and conduct in Bali. In C. Geertz (Ed.), The interpretation of cultures (pp. 360-411). New York: Basic Books.

Geertz, C. (1980). Negara: The theatre state in nineteenth century Bali. New Haven: Princeton University Press.

Geertz, C. & Geertz, H. (1975). Kinship in Bali. Chicago: University of Chicago Press.

Goldberg, S. (1977). Infant development and mother-infant interaction in urban Zambia. In P. Leiderman, S. Tulkin and A. Rosenfeld (Eds.), Culture and infancy: Variations in the human experience (pp. 211-243). New York: Academic Press.

Kestenberg-Amighi, J. (1990). The application of the KMP cross-culturally. In P. Lewis and S. Loman (Eds.), The Kestenberg Movement Profile: Its past, present applications and future directions (pp. 34-51). Keene, NH: Antioch New England Graduate School.

LeVine, R. (1977). Child Rearing as Cultural Adaptation. In P. Liederman, S. Tulkin and A. Rosenfeld (Eds.), Culture and infancy: Variations in the human experience (pp. 15-28). New York: Academic Press.

LeVine, S., & LeVine, R. (1981). Child abuse and neglect in subsaharan Africa. In J. Korbin (Ed.), Child Abuse and Neglect (pp. 35-55). Berkeley: University of California Press.

Lewis, M., & Ban, P. (1977). Variance and invariances in the mother-infant interaction: A cross cultural study. In <u>Culture and infancy: Variations in the human experience</u> (pp. 329-43). New York: Academic Press.

Marcus, G., & Fischer, M. (1986). <u>Anthropology as Cultural Critique</u>. Chicago: University of Chicago Press.

Mead, M. (1972). Personal communication.

Wikan, U. (1987). Public grace and private fears. <u>Ethos, 15(4)</u>, 337-363.

Wikan, U. (1989). <u>Managing Turbulent Hearts: A Balinese Formula for Living</u>. Chicago: University of Chicago Press.

The Essence of Gender in Movement

Warren Lamb

Introduction

The distinction between masculine and feminine movement is usually taken for granted, based on stereotypical assumptions about male and female behavior. Our culture associates rough and tumble play with boys, and caring for dolls with girls. Lore and old wives' tales abound regarding the appropriate expression of masculinity and femininity.

Physical differences also affect the perception of movement. The gender-specific distribution of muscle and fat in men and women influences movement. Also, secondary sexual characteristics (such as hair distribution) influence attitudes toward expression of gender. Interaction between the sexes is often judged in terms of its sexual connotations, as either heterosexual, homosexual, bisexual, or asexual. There has also been growing awareness of the effect of medication (particularly hormones) on sexual expression. As a result of these influences, it is difficult to separate gender, sexual identity and sexual preference from objective observation of movement.

All of this obscures the answer to the question of whether there are universal distinctions between movements of the two sexes. However, this question is important to raise now, as it may have great relevance in this time of changing sexual roles and challenges to traditional assumptions about gender.

Are Laban's theories relevant to this question? Can Labanotation scores show the difference between male and female movements? Can the Space Harmony Scales of Laban Movement Analysis be used to show these differences? If the answer to any of these questions is positive, can Laban practitioners provide understanding or direction for the shift in gender roles, particularly the emergence of women into a place of power in society?

While teaching at his Art of Movement Studio in the 1940's, Laban suggested that strong efforts were masculine and light efforts were feminine. He referred to the icosahedron A and B scales as, respectively, male and female. He used these assumptions to help train women who were filling factory jobs during the Second World War. For example, in a tire factory where men had used brute strength to lift a large tire, he taught women to do the same task, using a swinging movement instead (Laban & Lawrence, 1974).

A new approach to distinguishing between male and female movement is presented in this paper. It results from a search for the intrinsic differences — as free from cultural conditioning as possible — and is based on Laban's codification of movement. Thousands of randomly selected observations were made in Europe, North America, Africa, India and Southeast Asia, of men and women in streets, restaurants and other public places. Observations were recorded using a form of Labanotation. These observations were then analyzed in terms of two aspects of flow: flow of shape (growing vs. shrinking) and flow of effort (free vs. bound) (Figure 1). These flow variations were integrated with Laban's framework for observation of movement:

Shape (convex vs. concave): spreading vs. enclosing, rising vs. descending, advancing vs. retreating, and growing vs. shrinking.

Convex variations result in some form of opening of the body, while concave movements result in a relatively closed shape.

The use of the term Indulging is an attempt to describe movement which displays the common features of indirecting, diminishing pressure, decelerating and freeing, while Fighting describes the opposite bi-polar movement quality of focusing, increasing pressure, accelerating and binding.

Effort (indulging vs. fighting): indirecting vs. focusing, diminishing pressure vs. increasing pressure, decelerating vs. accelerating, and freeing vs. binding.

Figure 1. Flow of Shape and Flow of Effort

EFFORT

Indulging		**Fighting**
Indirecting	FOCUS	Increasing
Decreasing	PRESSURE	Increasing
Decelerating	TIME	Accelerating

Flow of Effort

Free	Bound

SHAPE

Convex		**Concave**
Spreading	HORIZONTAL	Enclosing
Rising	VERTICAL	Descending
Advancing	SAGITTAL	Retreating

Flow of Shape

Growing	Shrinking

The Flow of Shape

The flow of movement is crucial to the intrinsic attributes of masculinity and femininity. The concept of flow often appears in a non-physical or mystical context. We will concentrate on forms of flow which can be clearly observed. The two major aspects of flow will be presented and discussed separately, and then integrated.

The flow of shape refers to movement which increases or decreases the kinesphere. The kinesphere is the bubble of space surrounding the body, which circumscribes the limits of our reach. The possibilities for expressive actions within this sphere are referred to as shaping of space. However, shape-flow refers only to the shaping — growing or shrinking — of the kinesphere itself, regardless of what the person is doing inside it (Figure 2).

We can gain awareness of this process of growing and shrinking by concentrating on our breathing. With inhalation, we are inflated by the air and grow, becoming larger, with a bigger bubble of air in which to move. With exhalation, we shrink, becoming smaller, with a smaller bubble of air in which to move. However, the usual associations are not always true. It is possible to breathe out while growing in the flow of movement and to breathe in while shrinking. Nor is there necessarily any consistent link with growing and shrinking or the two processes of inhalation and exhalation.

This growing and shrinking can be clearly observed in children. From the moment of birth, a baby can be seen to expand and contract its kinesphere. At this age, these shifts are not yet directly associated with specific emotional states, but are a form of self-expression present at all times. Around age three, it becomes more feasible to associate growing and shrinking with emotional states, such as excitement and distress, respectively (cf. Kestenberg, 1975).

However, these associations do not necessarily help us understand shifts in shape-flow, because we have to observe the process of change itself, and not just the relative largeness or smallness. A large adult may have a relatively big kinesphere, but we can still observe a small shrinking movement when he or she feels deflated. This person's size will remain at the inflated end of the continuum, and may not

Figure 2.

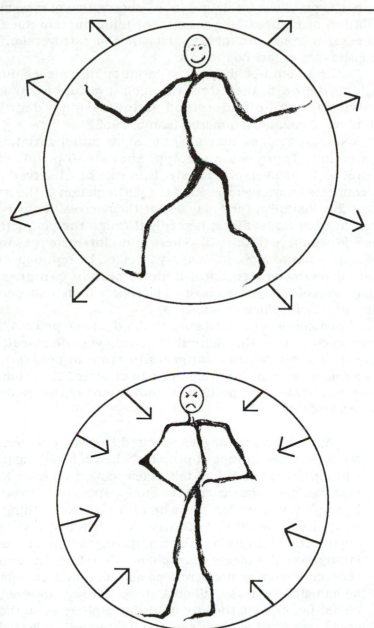

easily show changes in shape-flow. It is important not to apply simplistic psychological labels to the observation of movement. Inflation or bigness as a movement phenomenon does not necessarily imply confidence, arrogance or extroversion; the opposite may in fact be the case.

As the amount of shape-flow variation diminishes during childhood growth, the extent to which it occurs in an adult individual can be understood as indicating a degree of retention of childhood qualities (Lamb, 1965).

A small physique may also not show much variation in shape flow. There is a stereotype that small people often express themselves officiously; this can be observed as a disconnected movement lacking the participation of the whole body. For instance, they may assert themselves by thrusting their head or limbs disconnectedly through the perimeter of their kinesphere (Figure 3). There is no intrinsic reason for smaller bodies to move in this way . In fact, by repeated whole body growing movements, a short person can give the impression of occupying a bigger kinesphere than a tall person, without looking officious (Figure 4).

Movement is not a fixed state, but a dynamic process. This process continues throughout life (and even after death, in decay). When movement appears to stop, or ceases to be discernible, we have nothing more to observe. The following story illustrates the point that movement is the basis for expressiveness:

Mr. A, a general manager, admired the way his boss, Mr. X, handled groups of people: "when X is talking to a group, I have seen him take a few steps backward to maintain his distance from the group. This seems to set him apart as a leader, but when I try the same thing, people follow me!" Actually, X made a growing movement when he backed up, giving the group the impression of a bigger kinesphere. Therefore, the gap between them was not perceived as wider, even though he had stepped away. When A stepped away, however, he did not change the size of his kinesphere — so the group perceived a larger gap and instinctively followed him to maintain contact.

Figure 3.

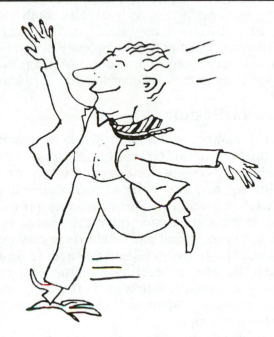

Figure 4.

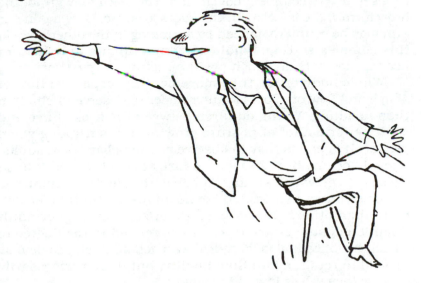

As can be seen in this example, the results of shape-flow changes will be affected by variables such as social status, cultural conditioning, and individual personality characteristics. Despite this complexity, it can be worthwhile to repeat this experiment in social settings, as it may help increase our awareness of growing and shrinking shape-flow.

Gesture vs. Posture

Partial body movement vs. whole body movement is another key distinction in understanding gender differences. A partial movement may consist, for example, of a shrinking movement involving the arm only: the arm will appear to occupy less space, as if withered. In a partial growing movement of the arm, the arm will appear to occupy more space, as if extended or stretched. In any partial movement there may be a tendency for the rest of the body to follow the arm. If the movement is isolated to the arm, it becomes a gesture (partial movement). If the movement is fully followed by the body (head, trunk and limbs all growing or shrinking together), it becomes a posture (whole-body movement).

An apparently simple outstretching of the arm may, in fact, be a set of very complex movements. The teeth may grind, the brow furrow, the fist clench, the knees lock, etc. Growing in one arm may be counterbalanced by shrinking in the other arm. In this complex setting, whole body movements only last for fleeting moments, in which posture-gesture merging occurs.

Whole body or posture movement in respect to flow of shape and flow of effort is much easier to observe in children than in adults. Young children between the ages of five and eight perform a lot of posture growing and shrinking when playing. It is not as easy to observe posture changes in adults. They do occur, but we seem to lose some of our childhood capacity to grow and shrink. Although the child's spontaneous responsiveness is modified, some adults retain this feature more than others. It has been theorized that higher adult retention of shape-flow flexibility is related to the degree to which the individual is identified with action. Such people may be said to retain a childlike quality, but do not necessarily express themselves in a childish way.

Shape-Flow in the Embrace

The above discussion of shape-flow, posture and gesture has been an introduction to understanding movement. In this paper, we will approach the topic of gender distinctions by observing and analyzing the movements involved in the act of embracing.

We can make a bold statement about most embraces, whether with the opposite sex, the same sex, between family members or between adult and child. If there is no involvement of posture (whole body growing or shrinking) the embrace will appear, to some degree, detached, aloof, or constrained. This does not mean that there is necessarily any less feeling in the embrace, that the embracer cannot otherwise be posturally expressive, or that other movement elements will not contradict this impression. However, based simply on the lack of posture, there will be some perceived lack of sincerity, effectiveness, or self expression (Winter, 1989). In some embraces, posture is present; in others, it is not (or only slightly present); and, some embraces are so complex that it is difficult to make any clear observation of movement at all. The following examples are offered as a rough guide to the kinds of embraces which typically involve posture involvement and those which typically do not:

Embraces With Posture Movement
- A parent embracing his or her child
- Lovers and potential lovers
- Old friends reuniting
- Good actors playing a romantic scene
- Boxers at the end of a fight

Embraces With Little or No Posture Movement
- A pre-occupied parent taking leave of their child
- Former lovers ending their relationship
- Political embraces
- Formal cocktail party greetings
- Older relatives (aunts, uncles) greeting dutiful younger relatives (nephews, nieces)
- Poor actors playing a romantic scene
- Boxers before beginning a fight

The Flow of Effort

In addition to shaping within the kinesphere, movement also involves the flow of effort. We use effort to get out of bed in the morning: effort gets us out of bed, while shaping dictates whether we fall on the floor or bump into a chair on the way to the bathroom. Rudolph Laban differentiated the effort component of movement from the shape component. The two are inextricably linked, as we can experience when getting out of bed, as well as in many other daily actions. An effort movement which is not accompanied by an appropriate shape movement will appear clumsy. A shape movement without an appropriate level of effort will appear listless.

Laban identified four effort elements, one of which is the effort element of flow, consisting of a polarity between bound flow and free flow. The variations between these two extremes occur along a continuum, which we can experience by altering our flow of effort from extremely bound flow to extremely free flow. Extremely free flow leads to abandonment of the body's structural rigidity, leading to a loss of balance if some degree of bound flow is not re-introduced. Extreme postural free flow looks ecstatic, spontaneous, free. It can be experienced by turning one's back to strong wind, allowing it to carry one forward. Extreme bound flow leads to complete rigidity; these movements appear highly controlled, directed, or tense. This extreme may occur in a person who becomes speechless with anger. Certain situations will usually cause us to emphasize bound flow, such as walking on a slippery surface, or across a narrow walkway with a big drop on each side (although it can be counterproductive to over-emphasize bound flow in these situations). Breathing also helps us experience this polarity: breathing out natually encourages free flow, while breathing in naturally encourages bound flow. However, as with shape-flow, it is possible to go against this natural tendency.

Observation of effort-flow in children reveals patterns that are similar to the developmental observations of shape-flow. When babies first learn to walk, they career along in a state of whole body (postural) free flow. When they fall and cry, their postural effort reverses to an extreme rigidity. The infant's whole body variation between free and bound flow is more extreme, and occurs much more regularly, than variations in an adult. As children grow and master other components of movement, we see a diminution in their use of flow of effort, as well as flow of shape. The impression of child-like responsiveness in some adults, which was mentioned earlier, is created as much by their immature patterns of effort flow as by their immature patterns of shape flow.

Observation of embraces in terms of effort-flow reveals patterns which are similar to those of shape-flow. When sincerity and shared emotion appear to be present, we see posture variation along the continuum of free and bound movement. When the embrace is superficial, formal, dutiful or unreciprocated, we see little flow of effort. This association may not be irrefutable, but it has been observed across a wide range of cultures.

A Framework of Shape and Effort

We can summarize this introduction to the four polarities of movement as follows:

1. Flow of shape appears as relative movements of growing vs. shrinking.
2. Flow of effort appears as relative movements of freeing vs. binding.

There is no physical reason why both genders should not equally use these four polarities of movement; and cultural conditioning is not relevant in the search for intrinsic qualities of movement by gender. Western culture has favored a growing expansionist posture as masculine and a shrinking demure posture as feminine, but this is now out-moded and there probably always have been exceptions. A man can shrink his kinesphere without appearing feminine and a woman can grow her kinesphere without appearing masculine. Similarly, men and women can both emphasize free or bound flow without necessarily taking on any attributes of the opposite sex. So far we have only introduced the parameters of movement, without linking them to gender attributes, in order to avoid any prejudice or cultural conditioning about the effects of gender on movement.

As a disciplined study, movement is still in the early stages of its development. One of its major difficulties is the lack of standard methods of observation, recording and analysis of complex body movements (film and video recordings assist in observation, but not in recording or analysis). These immense problems of definition mean that it is extremely difficult to communicate with confidence that there will be a consensus about what is being described. Furthermore, the lack of historical study of movement (other than dance) restricts the recognition of researchers.

Nevertheless, much progress has been made in addressing this problem, especially based on Laban's principles. Therefore, his framework of effort and shape movement terms is summarized and illustrated below. This framework cannot describe all movement, but does cover enough (when added to the elements of shape-flow and effort-flow already defined) for our purpose of analyzing gender-related movement patterns. This observational framework can be summarized as follows:

Shape
- Spreading vs. enclosing
- Rising vs. descending
- Advancing vs. retreating
- Growing vs. shrinking

Effort
- Indirecting vs. focusing
- Diminishing pressure vs. increasing pressure
- Decelerating vs. accelerating
- Freeing vs. binding

Relationship of Movement to Gender

Application of the above observational framework to movement according to gender reveals the following associations:

1. Women associate growing shape-flow with spreading, rising and advancing postural movements.

2. Men associate growing shape-flow with enclosing, descending and retreating postural movements.

Since movement can be more complex than the simple framework which we are using, it is also possible that no postural movement will be observed. These effects can be observed even in classroom experiments with a mixed group. However, let us observe them in an embrace between the sexes, and see what can be inferred. Later we will delve more deeply into the implications.

Women spread their arms to welcome men, growing and spreading simultaneously. It would appear to contradict their openness to simultaneously spread and shrink. However, men do not appear to feel this contradiction, as they apear to shrink with the spreading movement. It would appear that the more contained kinesphere gives them a greater feeling of control. As such observations have been made across cultures the tendencies would appear to be a relative preference and not culturally conditioned.

Men enclose women to them. In the process, they grow, shape their posture into a concave retreating movement, and may include a descending movement. It would appear that they want the bigger kinesphere to operate in, while feeling that the concave shaping (enclosing, descending and retreating) is necessary to receive another person. Women, however, appear to find it more satisfying to shrink as they enclose, descend and retreat (see #3 below). Perhaps women will grow at a later stage, probably with spreading, rising and advancing, (as in #1 above).

3. Women associate shrinking shape-flow with enclosing, descending and retreating postural movements.

4. Men associate shrinking shape-flow with spreading, rising and advancing postural movements.

If the woman draws away from an embrace, this could imply either a momentary interruption or a withdrawal from the embrace (shrinking). As she does so, she wraps her arms around herself (enclosing) and sinks into herself (descending). Her body shape, no longer convex and contained by the embrace, becomes concave (retreating). The man shrinks, and their formerly shared kinesphere separate from each other. As he shrinks, his body opens (spreading); he rises and advances.

The man shrinks his kinesphere, perhaps in order to maintain a bodily sense of control, and simultaneously spreads, to keep himself available for a new embrace. Although shrinking concavely, he also maintains a rising movement and a convex forward advancing potential. The woman's shrinking shows no such potential, as she shrinks, encloses, descends and retreats. Perhaps the man's instinctive sensing of this reinforces his advancing movement.

5. Women associate free flow of effort with directing (focusing) and accelerating postural movements, and increasing pressure.

6. Men associate free flow of effort with indirecting and decelerating postural movements, and diminishing pressure.

At this point, there is a hint of abandon in the man's movement, and his attention is all over the place (indirecting). His touch becomes lighter (diminishing pressure). Where he previously felt a sense of urgency, he now seeks sustainment (deceleration). As the woman's movement becomes more free, her attention is more focused. She gets firmer (increasing pressure) and becomes impatient (accelerating). If their kinespheres are in place, i.e., they are mutually sharing their growing and shrinking movements, the woman's movements may become more free. This requires her to direct her attention to her partner. Her touch pressure increases, to promote the free flow of movement, and her pace increases. As the woman's movements become more free, the man's are likely to become more bound.

7. Women associate bound flow of effort with indirecting, diminishing pressure and decelerating postural movements.

8. Men associate bound flow of effort with focusing, increasing pressure and accelerating postural movements.

The man focuses on controlling his movement toward his partner. He increases his force (increasing pressure) and speed (accelerating). The woman moves to reverse a movement tendency which leads towards abandonment (see #5). She becomes less focused (more indirecting), diminishes her pressure, and slows down (decelerates). As the man binds the flow of his movement he becomes more focused. He increases his pressure and acquires a sense of greater urgency (accelerating).

Summary and Conclusions

This description of an embrace is designed to give an impression of the movements involved. Although described in terms of relations between the sexes, these movement associations have primarily been observed in public embraces. These associations can also be seen in everyday behavior, even in embraces involving the same sex — and the opposite movement associations have not been seen. The embraces observed include these situations:

- Couples in parks
- Parents embracing their children
- Welcome and farewell greetings at airports, railway stations and other locations
- Stage performances

Within the complex interaction that takes place in an embrace, the following postural associations appear to be recurring tendencies in gender groups of diverse cultures:

Male
- Free effort-flow with indulging efforts
- Bound effort-flow with fighting efforts
- Growing shape-flow with concave shaping

- Shrinking shape-flow with convex shaping

Female
- Free effort-flow with fighting efforts
- Bound effort-flow with indulging efforts
- Growing shape-flow with convex shaping
- Shrinking shape-flow with concave shaping

Future Research

A distinct pattern has emerged from these observations, which is offered as a basis for further research. Experiments to test this hypothesis are difficult to set up because the subjects become self-conscious and lose the essential quality of whole-body spontaneity. However, the following experiments have been repeated with different groups:

I.
Have the group line up in a large room. Each person advances, in turn, across the room, as though he or she is being blown by a strong wind. The aim is to induce free flow of movement. If successful, people will progress in such a way as almost to lose control. About 3/4 of the way across the room, signal the person to assert bound flow (establish control). Have observers stationed at this point, to record the effort variations which accompany the transitions from free flow to bound flow, concentrating on whole-body movement.

II.
Have the group grow in shape flow as though to become airborne, like a balloon. Then, at a signal, everyone shrinks, as though his or her "balloon" has been pricked. Observers can record the shape variations which accompany the transitions from growing to shrinking.

It will be interesting to see whether others can confirm these associations, and feedback would be greatly appreciated. Comments are especially solicited in the following areas:

1. Observations by others: their apparent accuracy;
   how and when taken; whether the above
   associations were seen.
2. Exceptions.
3. Cross-cultural distinctions.
4. Means of separating culturally-conditioned behavior
   from intrinsic gender differences.
5. Suggestions for further research.

A Final Word

As mentioned earlier, the associations between shape flow and shape variations, and between effort flow and effort variations, were derived from observations objectively recorded in several parts of the world. No attempt is made to offer any interpretation of their implications beyond the suggestion that there may be a distinction — which transcends cultural conditioning — in the way that men and women prefer to move. In other words, is this distinction intrinsic?

References

Laban, R., & Lawrence, F. C. (1974). Effort (2nd ed). Boston: Macdonald & Evans.

Lamb, W. (1965). Posture and Gesture. London: Duckworth.

Kestenberg, J. S. (1975). Children and Parents. New York: Jason Aronson.

Winter, D. D. (1989). Empirical Studies of Posture-Gesture Mergers. Journal of Nonverbal Behavior, 13(4). pp. 207-223.

Body Movement and Cognitive Style: Validation of Action Profiling

Deborah Du Nann Winter, Ph.D.

Introduction

One of the most undeniable observations of nonverbal behavior is that people move their bodies (gesticulate) when they talk. Scientific attempts to understand these movements have for the most part focussed on their social value — the meaning that gesticulation adds to the verbal message which it accompanies. Thus, Ekman and Friesen (1969), drawing on Efron's (1941) earlier work, provided researchers with a valuable classification scheme of gestures based on the communicative functions of body movement: emblems and illustrators providing additional semantic meanings, regulators contributing to the structural organization of a conversation, etc. This approach has been so powerful that one often finds the field of nonverbal behavior equated with the field of nonverbal communication, and in psychology, the field of nonverbal behavior is usually seen as part of social psychology.

More recently, however, some researchers have suggested that body movement may have at least as much, if not more, to do with cognitive as with social processes. For example, Rime (1983) has argued that movement is the primary mechanism by which we come to perceive and understand our world, and that the intrapersonal process of articulating these meanings is aided by gesticulation. Here the focus is on the encoding rather than the decoding of meaning. Rimes' paper summarized many studies that fail to show a significant impact of nonverbval information on decoding accuracy, as well as other studies that show that restricting subjects' body movement interfered with their ability to organize and verbalize their meanings.

Focusing more specifically on the verbalization process, Freedman (1972, 1979) has also suggested that body movement facilitates the translation of thought into speech by helping the speaker focus on, and then symbolize, cognitive meanings. Thus body movement is necessary for the translation of thought into speech because of its focusing and representational functions. In a similar vein, Dittman (1972), noticing that gesticulation seemed to precede many verbal phrases, suggested that movement aids in planning or encoding them. Proposing a much more direct link between speech and movement, McNeil has postulated that gestures and speech are part of the same thought prosesses and that by observing them we directly observe the simultaneous inner speech (1982, 1985). Kendon (1986) has also argued along similar lines.

While not as frequently held today as the social view, the cognitive approach to the study of nonverbal behavor is certainly not new. In fact, the proposition that the study of nonverbal body movement is closely related to the thinking process has had a rich following in the history of psychology, endorsed by many important thinkers from quite diverse backgrounds. Structuralists (Wundt, 1973; Titchener, 1909), behaviorists (Watson, 1924; Washburn, 1930; and Skinner, 1957), Soviet psychologists (Sokolov, 1972; Kozulin, 1986), and cognitivists (Piaget, 1936; Werner and Kaplan, 1967; Bruner, 1968) have all, for one reason or another, supported this view in their theoretical arguments (Winter, 1989).

In light of the past frequency with which movement has been held as an essential feature of the origin of thinking, one is entitled to wonder why contemporary research on nonverbal behavior is so infrequently approached from the cognitive standpoint. Aside from the possibility that the field is still influenced by the Cartesian dualism which separates mental and physical functions, methodological limits may also play an important role. Perhaps, as several writers have argued (McGuigan, 1979; Lang, 1979; Cacioppo & Petty, 1981), we have only recently advanced our instrumentation to the point where we can electronically measure the subtle body movements which are associated with adult thought.

But another important methodological problem may be the difficulty of analyzing movement itself. Actually, the vast majority of nonverbal behavior research does not actually focus on movement, but on stable body positions such as postures and gestures (eyebrow lifts, eye contact, folded arms, nose wipe). This approach focuses attention on the result of the movement, rather than the quality of the movement itself. A movement-based approach would observe the movement quality with which the individual folded the arms, even if it didn't appear to result in any fixed state, or end-goal, and thus might be difficult to label. Unfortunately, until this point nonverbal researchers have lacked a viable model for analyzing and describing movement quality.

However, forty years ago, Rudolph Laban, a European dancer, choreographer, and architect, formulated several systems for analyzing human body movement (1950; 1956). He is best known in the dance community for his notation system, called Labanotation, by which many major modern dance works have been scored, similar to the way a musical composition is scored. For the most part, psychologists do not currently know his work, but when it is acknowledged, it is Labanotation that is usually referenced (Argyle, 1987). However, it is Laban's system of Effort Analysis (Laban & Lawrence, 1947) that is more useful for psychologists interested in nonverbal behavior, for two reasons: (1) Effort Analysis is scaled for the study of normally occurring body movement rather than dance and (2) Laban believed that effort qualities illuminate the thought processes.

While Laban generated the original insight that links body movement to inner processes, it has been his second and third generation students who have, with more precision and rigor, defined and formulated specific observation systems which can be used with various populations (Davis 1979; 1984; Kestenberg, 1975; Lomax 1967; 1968). One of the most accessible and intriguing of these systems was produced by Warren Lamb (1965; Lamb & Turner, 1969; Lamb & Watson,

1979), and refined by Ramsden (1972). Lamb was Laban's student and assistant in the early British factory studies which examined human effort during the Second World War. Lamb continued Laban's concern with Effort Analysis and elaborated it into the system now known as Action Profiling. Forty years later, Action Profiling is being used in management consulting: when business executives are interviewed, their body movement is notated, and information about their cognitive styles is then inferred from the movement data. The model assumes a relationship between movement quality and thought processes, such that the pattern of movements emitted during a two-hour interview can be analyzed to describe the individual's cognitive style.

While Action Profiling has been successfully used in management consulting, its basic tenets have not been subjected to formal empirical assessment. Affirming the validity of the Action Profile (AP) framework would illuminate one method of measuring a link between movement and thought. Perhaps validation might also contribute a viable methodology for studying the nature and development of the thought process as it relates to body movement. For these reasons, the purpose of the present work is to test the validity of the AP model.

Basic Principles of the Action Profile Model

Several features of the AP model need explication. First, AP focuses entirely on Posture Gesture Mergers (PGMs). PGMs are defined as moments when a posture (a full body movement) merges with a gesture (a movement of a body part) or vice versa (Lamb, 1965). These movements are formulated by Lamb as an indication of an authentic, healthy, involved expression (Lamb & Watson, 1979). Recent empirical work on PGMs supports this view; in a series of four studies, rate of PGM production was diminished by stress, deceit, frustration and perceived insincerity (Winter, Widell, Truitt, & George-Falvy, 1989). The authentic, healthy nature of integrated movement is also assumed by a number of movement/body therapy systems, such as Traeger, Feldenkrais, and Tai Chi (Juhan, 1987).

Table 1. The Action Profile Model

ASSERTIONS	PERSPECTIVES
(Effort Movements)	(Shaping Movements)

Stage 1: Attending

Investigating — making the effort to probe, scan, and classify information within a prescribed area.
Outcome: systematic research, establishing method, and defining standards.
(Movement = **space effort**)

Exploring — gaining perspective by perceiving the scope available, uncovering, encompassing, and being receptive to information from many areas. Outcome: creative possibilities, discovering alternatives.
(Movement = **horizontal shaping**)

Stage 2: Intending

Determining — making the effort to affirm purpose, build resolve, forge conviction, justify intent.
Outcome: persisting against odds, resistance to pressure.
(Movement = **weight effort**)

Evaluating — gaining perspective by perceiving relative importance, weighing needs, grasping issues.
Outcome: clarity of priorities, crystallizing issues, realism.
(Movement = **vertical shaping**)

Stage 3: Committing

Timing — making the effort to pace implementation, adjust to moment by moment changes in the situation.
Outcome: spontaneity, opportunism.
(Movement = **time effort**)

Anticipating — gaining perspective by perceiving the developing stages of action and foreseeing the consequences of each stage.
Outcome: setting goals, strategy.
(Movement = **sagittal shaping**)

When an individual's Action Profile is made, many body movements are ignored, and only the PGMs are counted. They are then analyzed in terms of six movement categories. Three of these are effort categories, which describe the dynamic quality of the movement in regard to space, weight, or time. The other three categories are termed shaping categories since they characterize the curvature of the body in horizontal, vertical, or sagittal planes. Each of the six movement categories is thought to accompany a cognitive process (Table 1). The assumption is that when engaging in these thinking processes, an individual naturally emits the accompanying movements. (One might theorize — Laban apparently did — that these cognitions are linked to these movements because of fundamental features of our physical bodies in geographical relationship to the world around us. (However, the present study will not examine the developmental aspects of AP). PGM profiles are believed to be highly stable over time after the age of twenty years.

Because of this stability, the pattern appears to indicate enduring features of the individual's cognitive style. The developers of AP posited that the individual's characteristic movement pattern indicates a deeply organized set of motivations to engage in certain cognitive operations. However, the model does not make statements about either ability or tendency to engage in these operations, since individuals can, and often do, engage in operations outside their movement pattern. But fragmentation of movement and eventual fatigue would be predicted to result from long-term activity outside the PGM profile (Lamb & Watson, 1979).

Testing the validity of AP is a multi-step problem, since several assumptions underlie the model. To guide the current research, three sub-questions were distinguished.

1. To what extent are the AP scores reliable? This question is similar to the generic question of consistency in movement style, which Allport and Vernon (1973) studied in their inquiry into the personality correlates of movement expression. If movement profiles are not consistent over time, judge, and condition, then it makes little sense to look for cognitive style implications of the profiles.

2. To what extent do movements and cognitive processes occur simultaneously? The validity of looking for long-term patterns of both movements and cognitive processes must rest on the fact that both are actually associated in a particular moment. That is, if it cannot be shown that different movement qualities actually accompany different cognitive operations, then it is pointless to look for enduring movement styles related to enduring cognitive styles.

3. Once the above questions are answered, then one can ask about the validity of associating body movement profiles with cognitive style. Ideally, movement profiles should be statistically associated with more than one measure of cognitive style. These considerations guided the following research.

The Measurement of the Action Profile

Since three of the following studies used AP scores, the procedure for scoring movement profiles will be generically described here. Any relevant variations from this procedure will be mentioned under each experiment.

All subjects were seated and interviewed for a minimum of two hours, during which their PGMs were observed and notated. The setting was a business office or conference room. The chairs were arranged so that the observers could see the full body of the subject. The content of the interview questions was not held constant, since it was believed that the scores would not be affected by interview content. (This assumption was tested in the first study). The interview topics ranged from work issues to any subjects that seemed to enhance PGM production. Interviews were continued until the interviewer recorded a minimum of 200 PGMs which were classified into six different movement categories (as in Table 1).

All movement profiles were scored by certified Action Profilers. Since many PGMs are small and distinctions between the six movement categories are subtle, considerable training is required before certification is granted by Action Profilers International. Certificaton is granted after the trainee's scores correlate at least .85 with a trainer's scoring of three consecutive subjects. Such agreement does not occur before the trainee has scored over 20 profiles under extensive supervision by trainers.

At the conclusion of the interviews, after the subjects had left, the interviewer calculated the profile scores by computing the percentage of PGMs which were observed in each of the six movement categories. (A number of other measures were scored as well, but they will not be described because they were not used in any of the following research). Scores were sent to the author, who subjected them to an arc-sign transformation before statistical analyses were run. This procedure corrected for the fact that the AP scores are percentages, and do not show a normal distribution (they tend to be positively skewed).

Experiment 1: Reliability of Movement Profiles

The purpose of the first study was to assess the consistency of AP scores over a variety of measurement variables (a condensed account of this study is described by Winter, 1987).

Method

Because AP has been used in management consulting for over 30 years, more than 5000 profiles are on file. In some cases, subjects were interviewed by more than one certified profiler for purposes of consultation among profilers. Selecting these subjects from the file enabled a test of various kinds of measurement error.

Subjects

Twenty-seven persons between the ages of 31 and 64 served as subjects in this study. Twenty subjects were British and American executive managers in mid-size to multi-national corporations, for whom Action Profilers had been hired as consultants. The other seven subjects were also British or American, and were either trained or training in Action Profiling, with considerable knowledge of movement analysis and AP techniques. There were three levels of subject sophistication:

1. Totally Naive: These subjects knew nothing about the AP method, and were recruited for the interview for "the purpose of some research" (n=5).

2. Semi-Naive: These subjects knew they were going to have a profile done, that it would measure their motivation, and that it had something to do with body movement, but were unfamiliar with AP assumptions, techniques, or scoring (n=15). Totally Naive and Semi-Naive subjects were all business executives.

3. Training: Subjects had various levels of training in AP and various degrees of familiarity with movement analysis and scoring implications. These subjects were primarily movement analysts and dance therapists (n=7).

Procedure

Interviews were conducted according to the description given earlier. Because subjects were culled from pre-existing files, it was not possible to evenly distribute subjects across measurement conditions. It was also not possible to tightly control measurement conditions; however, lack of such control in a reliability study is not viewed as a problem, but rather as a strength, since tight control can produce artifactually high coefficients. Naturally varying situations provide a more conservative test of reliability. There were three types of observation settings:

1. Simultaneous condition: Two judges observed the same subject at the same time.

2. Separate condition: Two judges observed a live session which was video-taped, and then another judge later observed the videotape. The time interval between different observations ranged from one day to seven and a half years.

3. Video/Live: One judge observed a live session which was video-taped, and then another judge later observed the videotape. The time interval between the video and live observation was at least one year.

Table 2. Reliability Coefficients for 27 Subjects (on Six Movement Categories) by Measurement Condition

Measurement Condition	Subject Sophistication			Mean
	Totally Naive	Somewhat Naive	Trained	
Separate Sessions	.87	.91 .81 .95 .81	.87	.88
Simultaneous One Session	.94 .80	.79 .81 .73 .98 .79	.90 .91 .84 .86 .84	.85
Video/Live	.85 .98	.91 .96 .98 .88 .78 .93	.88	.92
Mean	.89	.88	.87	.88

Similarly, there was no attempt to control the content of the interview, since it was thought that content would not affect profile scores. If the content did affect scores and was allowed to vary, reliability coefficients would be lowered, at least in the "separate" condition. Thus, comparing coefficients between "separate" and other"conditions would test the impact of content.

AP scores were independently completed by the interviewers, and then sent to the author, who calculated various measures of reliability. In all cases, judges were blind to other judges' scores.

Results and Discussion

Because AP scores are six percentages which sum to 100, they lack linear independence. To correct for codependence, correlation coefficients were computed on five of the six scores for each subject across judges, thus alleviating the determined score. In all cases, the last score was dropped before the coefficients were computed. Table 2 presents the resulting correlation coefficients, in terms of both subject sophistication and measurement condition. The number of coefficients in each cell indicates the number of subjects observed in that condition.

Coefficients ranged from .73 to .98 and averaged .88 across all conditions. Fisher Z tests failed to show significant differences between any of the mean cell coefficients, or between any of the row or column mean coefficients. Of special interest to the concern about interview content mentioned earlier, the mean of the separate sessions (.88) was not significantly or even numerically lower than the mean of the simultaneous sessions (.85).

These results indicate that scores on these six categories are consistent over time, modality (video vs. live scoring) and subject sophistication, as well as interview content. In all cases, reliability coefficients remained high, even when the interval between scores was 7 1/2 years.

Discriminant Reliability

Such consistently high reliability coefficients led to the question of whether judges were using the same scoring pattern and not discriminating sufficiently between subjects, thereby producing artifactually high coefficients. Several analyses were run to check this possibility.

First, the judges' scores were separated, then the mean and standard deviations were computed on each of the categories for each judge (Table 3). This data shows the degree to which judges were using similar scoring patterns across subjects. As Table 3 demonstrates, there does appear to be some

Table 3. Means and Standard Deviations of Movement Percentages by Judge

Space	Weight	Time	Horizontal	Vertical	Sagittal
Judge 1 (n = 12)					
M 20.25	21.08	15.08	20.25	10.16	13.16
SD 5.34	7.73	7.86	7.94	10.41	9.07
Judge 2 (n = 8)					
M 24.50	14.12	13.00	16.51	14.00	18.32
SD 6.88	5.59	8.24	8.71	11.36	11.00
Judge 3 (n = 4)					
M 17.25	12.50	20.75	14.50	17.25	17.25
SD 4.11	8.26	5.90	7.00	4.11	9.42
Judge 4 (n = 16)					
M 20.31	15.62	18.87	16.25	13.56	15.03
SD 6.31	7.41	9.24	7.60	7.88	8.27
Judge 5 (n = 10)					
M 18.60	16.30	18.30	19.30	9.32	18.18
SD 6.43	7.42	8.39	9.26	4.85	7.13
Judge 6 (n = 6)					
M 22.33	15.66	17.33	18.11	12.54	14.03
SD 7.17	6.62	7.47	10.55	9.62	10.03
Total 6 Judges (n = 56)					
M 20.58	16.48	17.08	17.92	12.05	15.89
SD 6.25	7.38	8.92	8.24	8.51	8.70

consistency across judges' patterns, since many judges give higher scores in the Space category and lower scores in the Vertical and Sagittal categories.

To assess the degree to which judges were prone to give the same profile, regardless of subject, a Kendall W coefficient of concordance was calculated between the scores of all subjects scored by each judge. It ranged between .11 and .35; this was not significant at the .10 level, but at the .20 and .30 levels, did show a tendency for judges to score subjects with similar patterns. However, this result does not tell us how these patterns affect the reliability coefficients, since in order to produce artifactual results, judges would have to use the same pattern, and these patterns would have to be used on the same subject. Two more analyses assess the likelihood of these possibilities.

To calculate the degree to which all judges' patterns are similar, a Kendall W coefficient of concordance was calculated on the rank ordering of judges' means for each movement category. This coefficient was .21, ($x2$ [5] = 6.30, p < .30), suggesting a small but nonsignificant overall homogeneity in judges' patterns across subjects.

In order to observe the degree to which this homogeneity actually impacted the reliability coefficents, an adjusted set of coefficients was computed. To remove the impact of judge patterns on subject scores, the mean of a judge's scores for subjects that the judge observed on that category was subtracted from each subject's score. For example, subject #1 was observed by judge #1 and originally given a space movement score of 23. Judge #1 observed 12 subjects and had a mean of 20.25 on the 12 space scores. Thus, subject #1 was reassigned a score of 2.75 (23-20.25) on the space category. All subjects' scores were similarly adjusted, yielding profile scores which were independent of judge patterns. Correlation coefficients were then calculated on the adjusted scores.

Table 4 shows the resulting data, which indicate very little overall impact of judge pattern on reliability scores. The mean of the adjusted reliabilities was .86 compared to .88 for the nonadjusted reliabilities. The adjustment lowered 15

Table 4. Reliability Coefficients Adjusted by Judge Scoring Pattern

	Subject Sophistication			
Measurement Condition	Totally Naive	Somewhat Naive	Trained	**Mean**
Separate Sessions	.82	.92 .85 .90 .86	.91 .82	.87
Simultaneous One Session	.86 .84	.84 .76 .86 .96 .77	.85 .96 .82 .92 .79	.92
Video/Live	.75 .92	.96 .91 .88 .81 .73 .94	.82	.86
Mean	.84	.86	.86	.86

coefficients, but raised 12, apparently because patterns which judges used on the same subject were sometimes dissimilar.

Thus, the conclusion from Experiment #1 is that judges can reliably score movement profiles and that, overall, they can discriminate well between subjects. In addition, scores are unaffected by subject sophistication or observation setting (video vs. live vs. simultaneous vs. separate).

Experiment 2: Movement Analysis of a Discussion Group

Method

The second study was designed to test the assumption that movement is simultaneously related to different thinking processes. To test the concurrent links between body movements and cognitive operations, a group discussion task was used. (Parts of this experiment are described in Winter & Goldman, 1987).

Subjects

Thirteen male and 16 female subjects between the ages of 18 and 38 participated in this study. None of them had any knowledge of AP. They were recruited by the experimental assistant,[1] and were for the most part her friends or acquaintances. Twenty-six of the subjects were students at a small private liberal arts college in the Northwestern U.S. The other three subjects were friends or colleagues of the author. Subjects were run in 13 groups of two or three people each. Each session lasted for approximately 90 minutes.

Procedure

Subjects met in the assigned room and were informed of the overall format and purpose of the experiment (no deception was used.). The study was described as an inquiry into the relationship between body movement and cognitive style, as demonstrated at various moments during a group discussion task. A videocamera (which was obvious) was pointed out and subjects were told that their discussion would be videotaped. An observer [2] was introduced to the group, and it was explained that she would go behind the one-way mirror to observe the group discussion from the video monitor. She would then join the subjects for a later segment of the experiment, when subjects would also have a chance to observe the videotape. Between segments, the author would teach the subjects a vocabulary to use in responding to the questions which the observer would raise while observing the tape with the subjects. Thus the experimental session was divided into three segments: 1) a group problem-solving task, 2) vocabulary instruction, and 3) data collection.

Group Problem-Solving Task

Subjects were told to rank a list of items that would be needed for a crash-landing of a rocket ship on the moon. The instructions were designed to elicit participation and sharing of ideas. Subjects were instructed to begin by ranking their choices individually, and then discussing their selections as a group in order to arrive at a consensus within 20 minutes. When the discussion began, the videocamera (Zenith model VC 1800) was switched to record mode, and a camera clock marked the videotape to within 1/10 second. While subjects discussed their lists, the observer watched the video without sound and listed camera times when a posture-gesture merger (PGM) occurred, as well as the movement category of the PGM (time, space, or weight effort; horizontal, vertical, or sagittal plane shape). Some movements had more than one category, so the observer chose the most dominant category for each PGM. Subjects worked for about 20 minutes, until they completed the task, or until the observer had listed at least 12 PGMs for each session.

Vocabulary Instruction

While the observer re-checked the tape and PGM categories, the author instructed the subjects on the six cognitive terms. Subjects were handed sheets defining Investigating, Exploring, Determining, Evaluating, Timing and Anticipating. Each of the terms listed synonyms, likely results, and verbal statements which would likely accompany such motivations (Table 5). The experimenter emphasized that the verbal statements were not necessarily the best guide, in that cognitive operations could occur with very different words being spoken, but that these statements might help subjects understand the way the experimenters were using various cognitive terms.

Table 5. Meanings and Possible Statements Accompanying Cognitive Operations in the Action Profiling Model

Process	Likely Results	Possible Statements
INVESTIGATING		
probing classifying defining questioning	points definitions questions distinctions	"What is the . . ." "Does anybody know what . . ." "What does . . . mean?" "How does this differ?"
EXPLORING		

broadening scope
changing scope
looking about
	ideas
	new slants
	different angles
		"What else?"
		"Is there an
		    alternative?"
		"Are there other
		    options?"

DETERMINING		

building resolve
amassing
    arguments
affirming point
	determination
	resolve
	justification
		"We should do . . .
		    because . . ."
		"We definitely need this"
		"This is more important"

EVALUATING		

weighing up
    issues
crystallizing point
ordering priorities
	issues clarified
	black/white
	    picture
	relative priorities
		"How does this
		    compare?"
		"The main point is"
		"This is more
		    important"

TIMING		

pacing
calming
seizing oppor-
    tunity
	urgency
	relaxation
	spontaneity
		"We need to get
		    started"
		"Let's hold off on this"
		"Since this is here
		    now"

ANTICIPATING		
foreseeing seeing trends seeing future/past	targets strategy structuring goals	"The long-range plan" "If this, then . . ." "First this, then . . ."

Data Collection

The observer and the video monitor were then brought in. Subjects were given answer sheets which listed the six cognitive terms for a series of at least 12 moments targeted by the observer. The observer then called out a time and a subject's name, and all subjects were instructed to watch the top left-hand corner of the video monitor to observe the exact clock time which had been called. Subjects were asked to try to put themselves "back into that moment" and then to select one cognitive operation from the six for the person whose name had been called at that clock time. The tape was often played three or four times until subjects felt certain of their answers. All subjects gave answers for all listed moments, so that at times subjects were estimating their own thinking process, and at other times they were estimating the thinking process of others.

Results and Discussion

A total of 166 PGMs were observed over the 14 sessions. Data were analyzed in three categories: Self Estimates, Other Estimates, and Combined (Self and Other). Since there were six choices for each trial, it was assumed that chance alone would result in a correct guess (hit) rate of 1/6 or 16.67%. A test for the significance of proportion was calculated. Table 6 lists the hit rates for Self, Others and Combined categories for each session, along with the average hit rate and Z score in each category. In each of the three cases, there were highly significant matches between movement and perception of cognitive operation.

For the purpose of this study, the data demonstrated a statistically significant link between operation and body movement. However, Table 6 shows that the hit rates averaged only about one out of three (Self = .27; Other = .30; Combined = .29). Several reasons for this low accuracy may exist. First, of course, the model linking movement and cognition may not be entirely accurate.

Or, the movement/cognition link might not lend itself to observation or verbalization in all cases. Several methodological

Table 6. Correct Estimates (Hits) of Motivation from Movement

Session	Self # of Hits	Self # of Trials	Self %	Other # of Hits	Other # of Trials	Other %	Self and Other # of Hits	Self and Other # of Trials	Self and Other %
Pilot	6	17	.35	13	34	.38	19	51	.37
1	1	11	.09	6	21	.21	7	32	.22
2	6	11	.55	10	22	.45	16	33	.48
3	2	9	.22	5	18	.28	7	27	.26
4	4	12	.33	4	12	.33	8	24	.33
5	2	13	.15	7	16	.44	9	39	.23
6	4	15	.27	9	30	.30	13	45	.29
7	2	10	.20	4	10	.40	6	20	.30
8	1	17	.06	6	34	.18	7	51	.14
9	5	9	.56	5	11	.45	10	21	.50
10	1	11	.09	2	11	.18	3	22	.14
11	5	8	.63	6	16	.38	11	24	.46
12	3	10	.30	3	21	.15	6	30	.20
13	2	13	.15	3	13	.23	5	26	.19
Total:	44	166		83	278		127	444	
Avg. % **(Correct)**		.27			.30			.29	
Chance		.17			.17			.17	
Z Score		3.33			6.00			6.0	
p<		.0001			.0001			.0001	

considerations relate to this problem, and could have hampered the accuracy of the ratings. Subjects had a very short training period, and instruction on the vocabulary may have been inadequate. Secondly, it may be difficult for subjects to distinguish cognitive operations, even when the vocabulary is clear. Subjects may have had difficulty remembering past cognitive events. In some cases, it seemed that the verbal statements actually misled rather than facilitated correct guessing, in that the labels given by the AP model do not always correspond to the lay use of these terms. Even though a short time period elapsed between the discussion and the data collection, perhaps an even shorter interval is needed for subjects to really remember their cognitive experience accurately. These two concerns, of course, would produce opposite modifications in the experimental procedure, since enhancing the training procedure would lengthen the interval between the cognition and the measurement of it. It may also be the case that the optimal interval was used, even though the hit rates were not high.

Interestingly, Table 6 shows that hit rates across sessions varied a great deal, indicating that some groups scored as low as 6% and others as high as 63%. Also surprising, was that hit rates for the Self category were not any higher than hit rates for the Other category. There was a moderately high correlation between the Self and Other hit rate for each group (r = .60). From this it seems reasonable to conclude that the ability to discern motivation from movement might be a general one across targets, but not across groups (perhaps not across individual perceivers). Future research on this issue would be helpful. It might also be useful to know how performance on this task compares to other measures of nonverbal decoding, such as the PONS test (Rosenthal, Hall, DiMatteo, Rogers & Archer, 1979). Finally, a more precise analysis of the cognition/movement relationship could in time answer the question of whether they are actually simultaneous, as McNeill (1985) and Kendon (1986) would predict, or whether the movement sets the stage for the thought process, and hence precedes the thought, as Dittman (1972) might predict.

Experiment 3: Concurrent Validation with
the Myers-Briggs Inventory

While experiment #2 showed a link between momentary shifts in body movement and the thinking process, the question of enduring individual differences in movement and cognitive style has yet to be addressed. The third and fourth experiments were designed to assess this question by studying ongoing patterns in personality and movement profiles.

Lamb (1965; 1979) has postulated that enduring PGM patterns indicate deep-seated motivation to perform specific actions within the profile. In his words, "the PGM pattern is a strong motivational force to particular behaviour. It has to be to expressed; we can repress it, but not all of the time, and so have an inbuilt compulsion to arrange our environment and circumstances for its expression" (Lamb & Watson, 1979, p. 124). Thus, AP scores should predict preferences for certain kinds of cognitive activities, as well as work and career choices. Experiment 3 examines the preference for activities, and Experiment 4 examines career choice.

To examine the link between AP scores and motivation for different kinds of cognitive operations, scores on the Myers-Briggs Type Indicator (MBTI: Myers, 1987) were correlated with AP scores.[3] There were several reasons why the MBTI was chosen over the myriad of other available personality measures. First, in its instructions to subjects, and in the wording of its items, the MBTI attempts to measure preferences, rather than talent, competency, adjustment, or lack thereof. Both the MBTI and AP profiles assume a neutral test situation in which the individual is free to express his/her natural inclinations. On both, scoring is designed to eliminate, or reduce as much as possible, evaluative connotations — that is, there are no inherently good or bad scores. Scores are designed to reflect an individual's preference for activities, given minimal situational constraints.

Secondly, the MBTI is focused on cognitive and perceptual processes. It describes the way individuals function in the

Table 7. Dimensions of the Myers-Briggs* as Applied to Work Situations

Extroverts	**Introverts**
Like variety and action	Like quiet for concentration
Sometimes impatient with long jobs	Can work for extended time on one job
Often enjoy talking on the phone	Dislike telephone interruptions
Prefer oral to written communication	Prefer written to oral communication

Sensing Types	*Intuitive Types*
Careful about the facts	May get their facts a bit wrong
Good at precise jobs	Dislike taking time for precision
Can oversimplify a task	Can overcomplicate a task
Reach conclusions step-by-step	May leap to conclusions quickly

Thinking Types	*Feeling Types*
Respong more to ideas than feeling	Respond more to feeling than ideas
Need to be treated fairly	Need to be praised occasionally
Tend to be firm and tough-minded	Tend to be sympathetic
May hurt others without knowing it	Enjoy pleasing others

Judging Types	*Perceptive Types*
Like to structure and finish jobs	Work best in fluid settings
Schedule projects efficiently	Work well under deadline pressure
May decide things too quickly	May delay decisions indefinitely
Use lists as agendas	Adapt easily to new input

*Adapted from *Introduction to Type* by Isabel Briggs Myers, Consulting Psychologists Press, 1987, p. 29. Coefficients were computed on raw scores.

world, "the way people prefer to use their minds, specifically the way they perceive and the way they make judgments" (Myers & Myers, 1980, p. 1). The concern is primarily with mental activity or cognitive processes, rather than with interpersonal traits, emotional, ego, or value functions which many other personality scales measure. Similarly, AP measures decision-making styles, and more specifically, the various preferences which result in different perceptual and judgment processes. Thus, both MBTI and AP are measures of cognitive style rather than personality style.

Finally, a recent flourish of MBTI use has been observable, and its application is increasing in a wide variety of settings. In spite of, or perhaps because of, its rather unsophisticated construction, it is one of the more frequently used scales today (probably because of its ease of interpretation and application). For these reasons, relationships between the two scales should be useful in further understanding the meaning of AP scores, provided that certain precautions are taken with the MBTI scoring, as described below.

Method

Subjects

Three sample groups of subjects were used for the present study. The first two were taken from data collected on management executives by Action Profilers at Nasser Associates by Schmikl and colleagues, as part of their management consultancy. This sample consisted of over 200 subjects for whom both AP and MBTI scores were collected as part of their interview program. These subjects were management executives in mid-size and multi-national corporations who were completely unfamiliar with both measures at the time of their collection. The size of this sample enabled a cross-validation check. By randomly splitting the sample in half, and independently testing all the hypothesized relations twice, the likelihood of spurious relations was reduced. Subjects who had some missing scores were deleted. This procedure yielded two samples, Sample A (n = 91) and

Sample B (n = 96).

The third sample consisted of 15 members of Action Profilers International who agreed to take the MBTI at a recent international meeting. Even though these individuals were very familiar with their AP scores (and could recite them from memory), they were not familiar at the time with the MBTI, or with various predictions formulated by the author (who was not present when the MBTI data were collected). Comparing the results of this sample with the results of the first two enables any effects of AP familiarity to be observed. Scores of all samples were sent to the author for statistical analysis.

Scoring Procedures

AP scores are percentages of PGMs, and hence add to 100. The MBTI, however, is scored quite differently. Table 7 lists major aspects of each of the eight preferences on the MBTI, particularly as applied to work settings, where AP scores are most likely to correspond in meaning. As Table 7 suggests, the MBTI assumes four independent bipolar dimensions with dimensions in the left column being inversely related to the dimensions in the right column. Thus, Introversion is the complement of Extroversion, Thinking the complement of Feeling, etc. MBTI interpretations are usually made on the basis of the "Type," a categorical label formed by the motivations with the higher score of each bipolar pair. However, this catergorical treatment of data loses much information about continual differences between scores. For the purposes of the present research, raw scores on each of the bipolar dimensions were used, resulting in eight Myers Briggs scores per subject. Use of raw, rather than scale, scores retained the maximum amount of information for these samples, while dispensing with the bipolar conceptualization, which AP scores do not use. All correlation coefficients were computed on raw scores.

Separation of Dominant Types

Categorical information on the MBTI is useful with respect

to the issue of dominant functions because it allows further tests of the AP model. For this reason, the three samples were further divided into dominance subgroups. According to the MBTI manual (Myers & McCaulley, 1985), preferences on the four dimensions interact in a dynamic way to produce dominance patterns. Dominance patterns refer to the primary dimensions of use and can be either perceptual (the Sensation vs. Intuition dimension) or judgmental (the Thinking vs. Feeling dimension).

When a MBTI is scored, feedback is usually given in four scaled scores, indicating the end of each of the four bipolar dimensions, and how far on each dimension the subject scored. Thus, a typical score might be I6 S21 T10 P14. This code means that the individual scored slightly higher on Introversion than on Extroversion, very much higher on Sensing than on Intuiting, moderately higher on Thinking than on Feeling, and moderately higher on Perceiving than on Judgment.

MBTI scoring practice specifies that (for various reasons stemming from Jungian personality theory on which the MBTI is based) individuals who show both Perception over Judgment and are Extroverted, use the perceptual dimension of Sensing-Intuiting (S-N) as their dominant function. Conversely, those who show Judgment over Perception with Extroversion use the judgment function of Thinking-Feeling (T-F) as their dominant function. The situation is reversed for the Introverts, who show T-F dominance if they have a preference for Perception over Judgment, and an S-N dominance if they show a preference for Judgment over Perception. Thus, the hypothetical subject above would be classified as a TF dominant because of the P and I combination.

In this manner, each of the three samples were further separated into two groups of dominance patterns. The samples were divided into SN dominant vs. TF dominant subsamples, based on the following criteria for their scale score differences (using scale rather than raw scores retains the most information because it sets the preference pattern relative to the larger samples on which the MBTI was normed):

S-N Dominant subsample:
>   Subjects showing Perception with Extroversion
>   Subjects showing Judgment with Introversion

T-F Dominant subsample:
>   Subjects showing Perception with Introversion
>   Subjects showing Judgment with Extroversion

This division allowed hypotheses of two different types to be tested: 1) those which deal with some general assumptions of the AP profile and 2) further tests of those which deal with specific relationships between AP and MB motivations. Hypotheses of the general type will be considered first.

Hypotheses and Results

For ease of explication, hypotheses will be described along with their rationale and results.

Concerning hypotheses about the general model, recall from Table 1 that AP scores are arranged in a 3 X 2 matrix which distinguishes three stages of decision-making (Attention, Intention, Commitment) along the dimension of Assertions vs. Perspectives (Assertions and Perspectives correspond to two types of movement information, Effort and Shaping movements).

The first test involves the decision-making stage, and proposes that dominance patterns will differentiate between Attention and Intention. In AP terms, the Attention stage refers to the gathering of information and ideas, and Intention refers to the basis on which an individual makes judgments about or organizes those ideas. In the MB model, Attention is similar to the perceptual function. According to the MBTI manual, Perception

> "includes the many ways of becoming aware of things, people, events, or ideas. It includes information gathering, the seeking of sensation or of inspiration, and the selection of the stimulus to be attended to . . . "
> (Myers & McCaulley, 1986, p. 12).

Similarly, attention in the AP model is defined as "actively prob[ing] . . . question[ing], . . . searching in order to find out

Figure 1. Predicted and Resulting Stage x Dominance Interactions

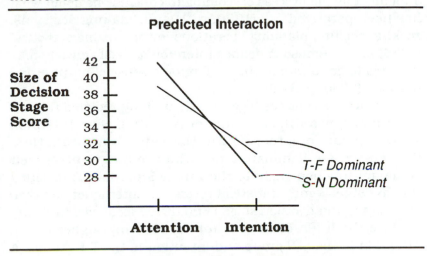

Predicted Interaction

Size of Decision Stage Score

T-F Dominant
S-N Dominant

Attention   Intention

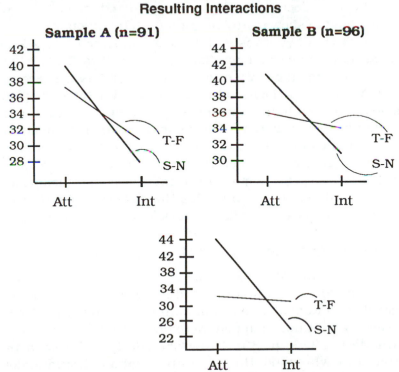

Resulting Interactions

Sample A (n=91)

Att   Int

T-F
S-N

Sample B (n=96)

Att   Int

T-F
S-N

T-F
S-N

Att   Int

On the other hand, Intention on the AP model is similar to the Judgment function of the MB model. Myers describes Judgment as the process of "coming to conclusions about what has been perceived . . . (1980, p. 1) and "making decisions, seeking closure, planning operations, or organizing activities" (1985, p. 14). Ramsden defines Intention as "self conviction. . . [coming] to grips with a job, . . . forging a sense of purpose and resolve." (1983, p. 34-5).

Putting these pieces together, then, it is predicted that SN dominant types will show higher Attention than Intention scores because perception is their dominant function. Conversely, T-F dominant types who use judgment as their dominant function ought to show more Intention. Translating this hypothesis into statistical terms, an interaction between dominance and decision stage is predicted as shown in Figure 1. Here the interaction is graphed, showing higher use of Attention in the S-N group and Intention in the T-F groups. A main effect for decison stage is also predicted, since overall, subjects tend to show more Attention than Intention.

To test this hypothesis, data were analyzed in a 2 X 2 analysis of variance with dominance type (S-N vs. T-F) as the first factor, and stage (Attention vs. Intention) as the second factor. As in each of the hypotheses to follow, the three samples allowed three independent tests. The results of each are graphed in Figure 1. Here it is clear that the hypothesis is confirmed, even though across all samples the Attention scores were much higher than Intention scores. In spite of this main effect, however, the proposed interaction is significant, as shown in Table 8, which includes the analyses of variance, along with means and standard errors for each condition.

Test of the Assertion-Perspective Dimension

The vertical columns of the AP model represent the distinction between Assertions and Perspective motivations. According to Ramsden, assertions involve "applying direct effort, making things happen, actively getting the job done" (Ramsden, 1973, p. 33). They are likely to be seen in individuals who make things happen, who act, and make

Table 8. Descriptive and Inferential Statistics for the Relationship Between Decision Stage and Myers-Briggs Dominance

Condition	Mean	Standard Error	Source	SS	df	Anova MS	F	p<
			Sample A (n = 91)					
ATT-TF	37.98	.82	Dominance	9.88	1	9.88	.28	.60
ATT-SN	39.09	1.01	Stage	2684.62	1	2684.88	77.10	.01
INT-TF	31.79	.82	StagexDom	113.33	1	113.33	3.25	.05
INT-SN	29.74	.86	Error	6190.71	178	34.73		
			Total	8998.55	181			
			Sample B (n = 96)					
ATT-TF	35.98	.93	Dominance	4.34	1	4.34	.09	.75
ATT-SN	38.51	1.03	Stage	1200.00	1	1200.00	27.37	.001
INT-TF	32.79	.87	StagexDom	2229.07	1	229.07	5.22	.02
INT-SN	30.87	.98	Error	8242.55	188	43.84		
			Total	9675.97	191			
			Small Sample (n = 15)					
ATT-TF	31.14	3.89	Dominance	26.25	1	26.25	.37	.54
ATT-SN	40.50	2.90	Stage	952.03	1	952.03	13.70	.001
INT-TF	27.85	2.64	StagexDom	418.00	1	418.00	6.04	.02
INT-SN	22.25	2.66	Error	1799.21	26	69.20		
			Total	3195.00	29			

changes in their environment. Similarly, Myers describes Extroversion as the ability to "get things rolling . . . (1980, p. 8) . . . to act on the environment, to affirm its importance, to increase its effect . . . to be action-oriented . . . " (1980, p. 13).

On the other hand, Introversion is described by Myers (1987) as "a thoughtful, contemplative detachment . . . a tendency to analyze the world, not to run to it . . . " (p. 23), "an interest in . . . concepts and ideas . . . " (p. 13). Similarly, Perspective in the AP model is described as "keeping things in balance, . . . seeing scope, . . . perceiving context, gaining awareness, and being less likely to act" (Ramsden, p. 33-34). Given these similarities, one would expect Introversion to be positively related to Perspectives and Extroversion to be positively related to Assertions. (Since the sum of Perspectives and Assertions must add to 100 in the AP model, they are absolutely inversely correlated. Therefore, there would also be negative relationships between Introversion and Assertions, and Extroversion and Perspectives.)

To test these hypotheses, Assertions and Perspectives scores were computed for all subjects by adding the appropriate motivation scores:

Assertions = (Investigating + Determining + Timing)
Perspectives = (Exploring + Evaluating + Anticipating)

Relationships between Assertions, Perspectives, Introversion and Extroversion scores were then compared, using Pearson product moment correlation coefficients. The resulting correlation coefficients are presented in Table 9. Although the small sample had too little power to demonstrate significance, the coefficients are in the hypothesized direction, and are clearly significant in the large samples.

Hypotheses About Specific Cognitive Motivations

The second series of hypotheses involve the relationship between MB scores and each of the six specific AP motivations. Each hypothesis was tested on each of the three samples; in addition, the dominance subsamples permit further tests. Tests will proceed from the top to the bottom of the AP model (Table 1).

Table 9. Intercorrelations between Assertion, Perspective, and Introversion and Extroversion

	Introversion	Extroversion
Sample A (n=91)		
Assertion	-.20*	.31***
Perspective	.21*	-.31***
Sample B (n=96)		
Assertion	-.36***	.28**
Perspective	.36***	-.29**
Small Sample (n=15)		
Assertion	-.40	.46*
Perspective	.40	.45*

*p<.05

**p<.01

***p<.001

Tests of Investigating

The first term is Investigating (upper left), which is defined as "defining, categorizing, fact finding, establishing method, teasing out information" (Ramsden, p. 34). Investigating is somewhat similar to Sensing on the MBTI. Myers and McCaulley (1986) define Sensing as "establishing what exists, realism, acute observation, memory for details" (p.13). In other words, both measure one's attention in the present, especially with regard to facts and details. These relationships should be even more strongly observable in that portion of subjects who use the perceptual function as their dominant function, the S-N subjects. Thus, the prediction can be tested by comparing

Investigating to Sensing in all three samples, and predicting that they will be stronger in the S-N subsamples of each sample.

The results showed that the correlation between Investigating and Sensing was significant at the .05 level in Sample A (r = .26, n = 91) and Sample B (r = .24, n = 96). In the S-N Dominant subsamples, the correlation was significant at the .01 level in Sample A (r = .31, n = 39) and at the .05 level in Sample B (r = .36, n = 43). In the small sample the correlations were not significant (r = .32, n = 15 in the full sample, and r = .48, n = 8 in the S-N Dominant subsample, although they were in the right direction.

Tests of Exploring and Timing

The next set of hypotheses relates to Exploring, which Ramsden defines as "having awareness, of scope, looking for alternative possibilities and approaches, questioning assumptions" (p. 34). Exploring is likely to overlap with two facets of the MBTI: first, Intuition, which Myers defines as "brainstorming, inspiration . . . , perception beyond what is visible . . . " (Myers & McCaulley, 1986, p. 12), "seeing new possibilities" (Myers, 1987, p. 5). Secondly, Exploring ought to be related to Perceiving, defined as "keeping open to possibilities . . . , curious, adaptable . . . " (Myers & McCaulley, 1986, p. 14).

Since the focus is the relationship between Exploring with both Intuition and Perception, it seems efficient to also propose here that timing ought to be related to both. Timing is defined as "sens[ing] . . . the appropriate moment, seizing opportunities, [being] flexible [with changes in] programming" (Ramsden, p. 34). In other words, timing is spontaneity. Myers describes Perceiving as "an ability to see the need of the moment and to turn easily to it . . . " (1986, p. 26) and Intuition as "inspiration" (1987, p. 5) ". . . leaping quickly to conclusions . . . " (1987, p. 29). Thus, the following positive correlations are predicted:

> Exploring with Intuition
> Exploring with Perception
> Timing with Intuition
> Timing with Perception

Table 10. Intercorrelations Among Exploring, Timing, Intuiting, and Perceiving

	Sample A			
	Total Sample (n=91)		S-N Dominant Subsample (n=39)	
	Exploring	Timing	Exploring	Timing
Intuiting	.28**	.34**	.45**	.37*
Perceiving	.24**	.41***	(test not possible)	

	Sample B			
	Total Sample (n=96)		S-N Dominant Subsample (n=43)	
	Exploring	Timing	Exploring	Timing
Intuiting	.24**	.23*	.31*	.19
Perceiving	.28**	.20*	(test not possible)	

	Small Sample (n=15)		S-N Dominant Subsample (n=8)	
	Exploring	Timing	Exploring	Timing
Intuiting	.37	.29	.41	.28
Perceiving	.35	.23	.37	.30

*p<.05
**p<.01
***p<.001

With regard to the dominance subsamples, it is only possible to test the hypothesis with Intuition, since Perception is used as one of the criteria for separating dominance subsamples. In Table 10 the results of these predictions are listed. In most cases, the predictions were confirmed with significance beyond .05. However, there are a few scattered exceptions, especially in the small sample where correlations of .24 through and .34 failed to reach significance, again probably because of small sample size. The only really clear disconfirmation of the hypothesis occurred in Sample B where the S-N dominant subsample showed a correlation between Intuition and Timing of .19. Unlike the general pattern across othe other two samples, the S-N dominant subsample of Sample B did not show higher correlations than the full Sample B. However, for the most part, the hypotheses were confirmed, showing significant positive coefficients in 11 of 12 cases with sufficient power.

Test of Determining, Evaluating and Anticipating

Three AP motivations, which will be considered separately, overlap with the MB Judging function: Determining, Evaluating, and Anticipating. Ramsden defines Determining as "having firmness of purpose, determination, persistence against difficult odds, resistance to pressure, strong conviction" (1973, p. 34). Similarly, Myers describes Judging as appearing "organized, purposeful, and decisive . . . " (Myers & McCaulley, 1986, p. 14). Judging should also overlap with Evaluating, which is defined as "crystallizing issues, establishing importance, challenging; [having] realistic recognition of immediate needs; forthright acceptance of hard facts" (1973, p. 34). Judging should also correlate with Anticipating, defined as "looking ahead, farsightedness, foreseeing consequences of action; evaluating future programming" (Ramsden, 1973, p. 34). With respect to Anticipating, Judging is described as "scheduling projects so that each step gets done on time" (Table 5). Thus, positive relationships between Judging and Determining, Exploring, and Anticipating were predicted.

Table 11 shows the resulting coefficients, which support the predictions. Judging was significantly related to all three

Table 11. Intercorrelations of Judging with Determining, Evaluating, and Anticipating

	Determining	Evaluating	Anticipating
Sample A (n = 91)			
Judging	.24*	.22*	.27*
Sample B (n = 96)			
Judging	.34***	.31**	.22*
Small Sample			
Judging	.36	.26	.30

*p < .05
**p < .01
*** p < .001

AP motivations in the two large samples; although again, lack of power in the small sample resulted in no significance.

Discussion and Conclusion

Figure 2 summarizes the various hypotheses and their tests in terms of the AP model. Each of the AP terms are shown with their predicted relationship to MBTI measures. Note that even though some AP measures have similar postulated relationships to MBTI scores, each AP term has a unique combination of hypothesized relationships to the MBTI measures. As a series of observations, the data support a large number of predictions relating the MBTI to AP scores. The fact that three independent samples were used to test each prediction enhances the confidence we may place in these coefficients.

Since many predictions were tested in this study, the data were re-examined raising the alpha level to .01, thereby reducing the likelihood of Type I error. With this more conservative criterion, 17 of the 47 predictions show statistical significance. These results are supportive of the hypotheses only if nonpredicted relationships show a weaker significance rate. To address this question, all other possible relationships were calculated. Six subscales on the AP measure and eight subscales on the MBTI were intercorrelated for each of the three samples, bringing the total number of possible correlations to 144. (For the sake of simplicity, dominance

Figure 2: Summary of Tested AP-MBTI Relationships

	Assertion **Extroversion**	**Perspective** **Introversion**
Attention **S-N**	Investigating Sensing	Exploring Perceiving Intuiting
Intention **T-F**	Determining Judging	Evaluating Judging
	Timing Intuiting Perceiving	Anticipating Judging

subsamples were not used in the following analysis). Since there were 34 predicted relationships, 110 were not predicted. Of these 110, only five reached significance at the .01 level, and another one at the .05 level. None of these six significant coefficients generalized across samples or measures. Clearly, the success of the predicted relationships cannot be attributed to low discriminant validity.

However, no matter how strong the results of this study, it is still a paper-and-pencil test, subject to all the limitations of this kind of measure, including the concern that the MBTI may be a particularly transparent individual difference questionnaire. A more convincing demonstration of AP validity might come from comparing scores to a richer measure of behavior. For this reason, the last study in this series compared profile scores of different professional groups.

Experiment 4: Contrasted-Groups Design

If AP describes meaningful differences in cognitive style, it ought to differentiate between different occupational groups. Earlier it was stated that PGM profiles are not meant to illuminate ability or achievement in certain cognitive operations, since individuals can and do operate outside of their profiles quite frequently. However, it would not be expected that persons operating for long periods of time outside of their profiles would feel fulfilled by that activity, since fragmentation would eventually lead to stress and fatigue. For this reason an attempt was made to choose subjects in this study who had worked in their field for ten years, and felt fulfilled by that work.

Method

Subjects

Subjects consisted of professional adults (51 male and nine female) between the ages of 26 and 62. They were British, Canadian, and American citizens, and were interviewed in their country of residence.

Occupational groups were chosen for the kind of cognitive process required by each profession. Six groups were selected because each group should score high on one of the six different cognitive processes in the AP model (Table 1). Thus:

1. Accountants were chosen because they should score high in Investigating (indicated by Space Effort movements). Investigating is probing, working with details, classifying information, and establishing systematic method.
2. Inventors were chosen because they should score high in Exploring (Horizontal Shaping movements). Exploring is looking for alternatives, widening the scope available, and discovering creative possibilities.
3. Barristers (courtroom lawyers) were chosen because they should score high in Determining (indicated by

Weight Effort movements). Determining is affirming and reaffirming purpose, building resolve, persuading others, and resisting pressure.

4. Historians were chosen because they should score high Evaluating (indicated by Vertical Shaping movements). Evaluating is clarifying issues, perceiving relative importance, and crystallizing principles underlying many items.

5. Salespersons were chosen because they should score high in Timing (indicated by Time Effort movements). Timing is pacing implementation, adjusting to immediate situational demands, and acting at opportune moments.

6. Chess players were chosen because they should score high in Anticipating (indicated by Sagittal Shaping movements). Anticipating is foreseeing consequences and planning sequence of actions, thinking in if/then contingencies, and setting future goals.

Subject recruitment

Subjects were recruited in a variety of ways. Two of the groups (Accountants and Salespersons) were taken from the existing file of 5000 profiles mentioned in Experiment 1. All subjects fit the criteria of having worked in their field (accounting or sales) for at least ten years. Profiles were drawn from the 5000-subject file by a clerk who was asked to submit ten profiles in each category; the clerk was completely unfamiliar with the nature of the research, or any of its hypotheses. (In these groups, it was not possible to check the level of fulfillment which subjects felt about their work.)

Other groups were recruited by certified Action Profilers[4] who volunteered to help collect data for a research project. Subjects were contacted and asked to participate in a research study which would involve a two-hour videotaped interview. In some cases, the profiler knew the subject personally, and so was able to secure participation, as well as names of associates who might also be willing to participate. Subjects were offered the opportunity to get feedback on their interview, if they so desired.

Other features of each occupational group will be described separately: Inventors were recruited from the New York City area, and all belonged to an organization whose membership was limited to those holding patents on "intellectual property." Although not all felt they were financially successful, all had been inventing for at least ten years and enjoyed the work. Barristers were recruited from the London area and had been practicing courtroom law for at least a decade. Historians were all American or Canadian Ph.D.'s or Ph.D. candidates. They included academics as well as several museum curators. Five of the historians were graduate students and had been working in history for a minimum of five, rather than ten years. (Recruitment of this category was difficult, and since less time in the field would only create a more conservative test of the hypothesis, the criterion for subject selection was lowered for this group). Finally, the chess players were all American or Canadian and had American ratings in chess (a measure of playing effectiveness) of at least 2000. Many were members of a chess club in Manhattan.

Control for experimenter effect

Since data collectors knew some of the subjects personally, and most knew at least something about the hypotheses, control for experimenter effects is crucial to the interpretation of this experiment. Unfortunately, it was not possible to keep all data collectors blind to all conditions, since occupational membership would be obvious in the interview. Instead, a system of blind observation was randomly distributed over the design. Most interviews were taped, and 27 taped interviews were sent to a blind reviewer, who scored the interviews without sound, and thus, without knowledge of group memberships.[5] In all cases, the scores of this blind reviewer were the scores which were used in the data analysis (rather than the scores of the original interviewer).

In addition, the scores of the accountants and salespersons were culled from pre-existing files by a clerk who was blind to the experimental hypotheses. Together, the scores of the blind judge and the blind clerk totaled 47 of 60 total scores analyzed in this study. To assess the likelihood that the remaining 13 scores could have been affected by experimenter expectancy,

Table 12. Means and Standard Deviations for 6 Occupational Groups on 6 Movement Categories

	Space	Horizontal	Weight	Vertical	Time	Sagittal
Accountants						
M	.27	.11	.16	.12	.18	.16
SD	.07	.07	.18	.08	.14	.08
Inventors						
M	.24	.24	.18	.06	.08	.13
SD	.03	.04	.07	.02	.04	.16
Barristers						
M	.21	.09	.24	.17	.17	.13
SD	.04	.04	.03	.07	.05	.04
Historians						
M	.22	.11	.16	.18	.20	.15
SD	.05	.05	.04	.06	.05	.09
Salespersons						
M	.07	.23	.16	.13	.26	.14
SD	.06	.10	.11	.15	.06	.10
Chess Players						
M	.21	.15	.18	.13	.19	.15
SD	.08	.09	.08	.09	.06	.08
Pool of Other 5 Groups						
M	.21	.15	.18	.13	.20	.15
SD	.08	.09	.08	.09	.06	.08

eight of the blind reviewer's subjects who had two sets of scores were correlated and the resulting Pearson Product Moment Coefficient was .90. This high inter-judge consistency converges with the results of Experiment 1, and makes the likelihood of experimenter effects operating in this design very small. Furthermore, this result reduces the likelihood that content or subject matter of the interview (which certainly was confounded with experimental groups) had an impact on the AP scores.

Results and Discussion

The means and standard deviations for each occupational group on each of the six profile subscores is presented in Table 12. To test the prediction that each occupational group showed a higher mean on its hypothesized particular cognitive process than did other groups, a 2 X 6 mixed model analysis of variance was run on each of the six dependent variables.[6] The two-level between-subjects factor was group membership. Each group was compared to the pooled mean of the other five groups. The six-level within-subject factor was the six subscales of the AP profile. In this design, interactions were predicted such that the occupation in question would show a higher subscale mean than the pooled mean of the other five groups on the predicted cognitive operation. Table 13 shows the resulting F values for each of the predicted relationships. These results clearly demonstrate significance for each of the predictions.

In addition, several other nonpredicted interactions appeared significant. Compared to the mean of the other five groups, Inventors showed significantly higher vertical movement counts (Evaluating); Barristers showed significantly higher time movement counts (Timing); and Salespersons showed higher space movement counts (Investigating).

General Discussion

Overall, the results of the four experiments support the validity of the AP scores as a reflection of ongoing cognitive style. The AP profiles appear to be reliable over time, judge, and observation situation, as well as meaningfully related to other measures of cognitive style, including the MBTI and

Table 13. ANOVA Tests for Each Occupational Group Against Pooled Mean of Other 5 Groups

	SS	df	MS	F	p<
Accountants on Investigating	.061	1	.061	21.672	.001
Inventors on Exploring	.101	1	.101	23.317	.001
Barristers on Determining	.046	1	.046	8.39	.005
Historians on Evaluating	.036	1	.036	5.05	.029
Salespersons on Timing	.053	1	.053	19.239	.001
Chess Players on Anticipating	.039	1	.039	6.419	.014

occupational group. Experiment 2 also showed the predicted relationship between body movement quality and simultaneous cognitive activity.

While the studies as a whole provide good preliminary support for the validity of AP, they only begin the inquiry into the theoretical relationship between body movement and cognitive operation. One issue that needs rather immediate attention is the role of language in linking the thought process to body movement quality. AP scores are primarily based on movements which individuals generate as they are speaking. People move more when they speak than when they think without speaking. In fact, nonvocalized thinking often seems to be accompanied by stillness, rather than movement. Would the more recent methodologies of measuring covert speech and subtle body movement with electric rather than visual data (McGuigan, 1979; Lang, 1979; Cacioppo & Petty, 1981) confirm the AP model when outward speech is not involved? Or is AP really measuring the process of translating thought into speech? If that is so, the role of language would seem to be pivotal, and AP might be regarded as a psycholinguistic rather than a cognitive measure. The author's current view is that AP measures a cognitive (intrapersonal) rather than a social (interpersonal) process because for the most part PGM quality is not decoded by listeners (unless highly trained). However, to the extent that AP is tied to verbal expression, a paradigm of social process becomes relevant, and AP may indeed be an example of nonverbal communication, rather than of simply nonverbal behavior. This is the position which Kendon takes in considering the close tie between gesticulation and speech (1986), arguing against McNeil (1985), who views gestures as more a matter of cognition and less a matter of social communication.

The studies reported in this article are meant to answer the question as to whether AP might provide a useful method for study of the motoric elements of human thought process. AP appears to meet traditional standards for reliability and validity, and so may well be a useful tool for scientists interested in pursing the relationship between movement and thought. However, questions about a tool's adequacy do not address questions about its accessibility. Currently, considerable training is required to learn how to distinguish the subtle qualities of body movement which AP measures. Since this training includes basic features of management consultancy (where AP is commercially used), some of it is not relevant for the scientist. The observation training needs to be gleaned and clearly formulated for scientists. Perhaps learning smaller components of the system for more specific research programs would be possible.

The aim of this research has been to present a number of investigations broad enough to answer the general question about the adequacy of the AP as a measurement tool; to the extent that the work is broad, it is also preliminary. Initial demonstrations of these phenomena only seem to open many more questions which deserve more careful and rigorous study. In this last section, some of the possible questions which can be addressed with the AP measure will be sketched.

For example, Experiment 1 demonstrates the reliability of

AP scores, but leaves unanswered questions about how and why movement profiles stabilize over time. Allport and Vernon's classic studies on movement consistency reached the same conclusions with the same unanswered questions over 50 years ago. Very useful in this regard is the fertile work of Kestenberg and her colleagues (1975; Kestenberg & Sossin, 1979) who use Laban based effort/shape analysis to study the personality development of infants and children. It would be helpful to know, for example, if AP scores are associated with stages of cognitive development, with intellectual development as measured by IQ tests, or with the genesis of symbolic processes. If Piaget and other organismic theorists such as Bruner (1968) and Werner and Kaplan (1967) are correct, thought develops originally from body movement. But how and why does body movement quality impede or facilitate the development of cognitive operations? In fact, from what bodily experience does human thought derive? Was Laban correct when he postulated that such movements arise from our geometric relationship with space?

Similarly, Experiment 2 demonstrates the viability of observing thought process from body movement quality but leaves many questions unanswered. Why are individuals not better at observing their own thought process than they are at inferring it in others? Does language which describes the thinking process hurt more than it helps? Should some labels in the AP model be changed so as to more adequately reflect the process? What abilities are required to accurately infer the thought process from the movement experience? Is this approach a return to the older question of introspection, or is basing the inquiry on objectively verifiable movement data a solution to the pitfalls of introspection?

While Experiment 3 clearly links AP meanings and MBTI meanings, the question remains how to best describe these individual differences. Are other measures of cognitive style a more useful way of framing these differences? Would a movement profile be a more viable way of describing differences than personality measures, which often rely so heavily on the semantic and socially approved meanings of the culture? For that matter, to what extent are the movement profiles culturally specific? What is the heritability of both movement and cognitive style?

Finally, if profiles can be used to distinguish occupational groups, could they be used to counsel individuals in career choice? What other kinds of practical problems might be addressed with a tool which measures a deeply organized pattern of cognitive and movement style?

These questions are far-reaching, but so might be the implications of the central finding here: that human movement and thinking are knit together, and that it may be possible to examine the latter by closely observing the former.

Author's Note

Parts of this research were supported by the Aid to Faculty Scholarship Fund, Whitman College. This work was designed and written solely by the author. Many individuals helped with data collection for various experiments and their assistance is gratefully acknowledged within the context of each study. Requests for reprints should be sent to Deborah Du Nann Winter, Department of Psychology, Whitman College, Walla, Walla, Washington, 99362.

Footnotes

[1] Carla Widell was the experimental assistant for this study.

[2] Ellen Goldman was the observer for this study.

[3] Much of the following description is taken from Winter & Schmikl, 1988.

[4] The author would like to express deep appreciation for the generous time and energy of the following Action Profilers who served as data collectors: Edward Bows, Ellen Goldman, Warren Lamb, Reena Liberman, Lynn McGregor, Pamela Ramsden, Kevin McGarrigle-Schlosser, Patricia Walker, Anastacia Gourley, Jody Zacharis, and particularly to Jane Maloney, who also coordinated data collection.

[5] The author is very grateful to Ellen Goldman for serving as the blind observer for this study.

as the blind observer for this study.

[6] The author would like to thank Scott Lewis for his help in running this analysis.

References

Allport, G. W., & Vernon, P. E. (1933). Studies in expressive movement. New York: Macmillan.

Argyle, M. (1987). Bodily communication. London: Methuen.

Bruner, J. (1968). Processes of cognitive growth: Infancy. (Vol. 3, Heinz Werner Lecture Series). Worcester, MA: Clark University Press.

Cacioppo, J. T., & Petty, R. E. (1981). Electromyograms as measures of extent and affectivity of information processing. American Psychologist, 36, 441-456.

Davis, M. (1979). Laban analysis of nonverbal communication. In S. Weitz (Ed.). Nonverbal communication: Readings with commentary (2nd ed., pp. 182-206). New York: Oxford University Press.

Davis, M. (1984). Nonverbal behavior and psychotherapy: process research. In A. Wolfang (Ed.), Nonverbal behavior: Perspectives, applications, intercultural insights (pp. 203-228). Lewiston, NY: C. J. Hogrefe.

Davis, M., Weitz, S., & Culkin, J. (1980). Sex differences in movement style: A multivariate analysis of naive and Laban-based ratings. American Journal of Dance Therapy, 3, 4-11.

Dittman, A. T. (1972). The body movement-speech rhythm relationship as a cue to speech encoding. In A. W. Siegman & B. Pope (Eds.). Studies in dyadic communication (pp. 135-151). New York: Pergamon Press.

Efron, D. (1941). Gesture and environment. New York: King's Crown Press.

Ekman, P., & Friesen, W. V. (1981). The repertoire of nonverbal behavior categories: Origins, usage, and coding. In A. Kendon (Ed.), Nonverbal communication, interaction and gesture. (pp. 67-105). The Hague: Mouton. (Reprinted from Semiotica, 1969, 1, 49-98).

Freedman, N. (1972). The analysis of movement behavior during the clinical interview. In A. Siegman & B. Pope (Ed.), Studies in dyadic communication (pp. 153-175). Oxford: Pergamon.

Freedman, N. (1977). Hands, words, and mind: On the structuralization of body movements during discourse and the capacity for verbal representation. In N. Freedman & S. Grand (Eds.), Communicative structures and psychic structures (pp. 109-132). New York: Plenum.

Juhan, D. (1987). Job's body: A handbook for bodywork. Barrytown, NY: Station Hill Press.

Kendon, A. (1980). Gesticulation and speech: Two aspects of the process of utterance. In M. Key (Ed.), Nonverbal communication and language (pp. 207-288). The Hague: Mouton.

Kendon, A. (1983). Gesture and speech: How they interact. In J. M. Wieman & R. P. Harrison (Eds.), Nonverbal interaction. Beverly Hills, CA: Sage Publications.

Kendon, A. (1986). Some reasons for studying gesture. Semiotica, 62, 3-28.

Kestenberg, J. S. (1975). Children and parents: Psychoanalytic studies in development. New York: Jason Aronson.

Kestenberg, J. S., & Sossin, K. M. (1979). The role of movement patterns in development, II. New York: Dance Notation Bureau Press.

Kozulin, A. (1986). The concept of activity in Soviet psychology. American psychologist, 42, 264-274.

Laban, R. (1980). The mastery of movement. Plymouth, England: Macdonald & Evans. (Original work published 1950)

Laban, R., & Lawrence, F. C. (1974). Effort: Economy in movement. Boston: Plays, Inc. (Original work published 1947)

Lamb, W. (1965). Posture and gesture. London: Gerald Duckworth.

Lamb, W., & Turner, D. (1969). Management behavior. London: Gerald Duckworth.

Lamb, W., & Watson, E. (1979). Body code: The meaning in movement. London: Routledge & Kegan Paul.

Lang, P. J. (1972). A bio-informational theory of emotional

imagery. Psychophysiology, 16, 495-512.

Lomax, A. (1967). The good and beautiful in folksong. Journal of American folklore, 80, 213-35.

Lomax, A. (1968). Folk song style and culture. Washington, DC: American Association for the Advancement of Science, Washington, D.C.

McNeill, D. (1985). So you think gestures are nonverbal? Psychological review, 92, 350-371.

Moore, C. L. (1982). Executives in action: A guide to balanced decision-making in management. Plymouth, England: MacDonald and Evans.

Myers, I. B. (1987). Introduction to type. Palo Alto, CA: Consulting Psychologists Press.

Myers, I. B., & McCaulley, M. H. (1986). Manual: A guide to the development and use of the Myers-Briggs Type Indicator. Palo Alto, CA: Consulting Psychologists' Press.

Myers, I. B., & Myers, P. B. (1980). Gifts differing. Palo Alto, CA: Consulting Psychologists Press.

Piaget, J. (1951/1936). The origin of intelligence in the child. (Margaret Cook, Trans.) Middlesex, England: Penguin. (Originally published in 1936 as La Naissance de l'intelligence chez l'enfant.)

Piaget, J. (1962). Play, dreams and imitation in childhood (C. Gattegno and F. M. Hodgson, Trans.). New York: Norton.

Ramsden, P. (1973). Top team planning: A study of the power of individual motivation in management. London: Cassell/Associated Business Programmes.

Rimes, B. (1983). Nonverbal communication or nonverbal behavior? Towards a cognitive-motor theory of nonverbal behavior. In W. Doise & S. Moscovici (Eds.), Current issues in European social psychology (Vol. 1). Cambridge: Cambridge University Press.

Rosenthal, R., Hall, J. A., DiMatteo, M. R., Rogers, L., & Archer, D. (1979). Sensitivity to nonverbal communication: The PONS test. Baltimore: Johns Hopkins University Press.

Sokolov, A. N. (1972). Inner speech and thought. New York: Plenum Press.

Skinner, B. F. (1957). Verbal behavior. New York: Appleton-Century Crofts.

Titchener, E. B. (1909). Lectures on the experimental

psychology of the thought-processes. New York: Macmillan.

Washburn, M. F. (1930) A system of motor psychology. In C. Murchison (Ed.), Psychologies of 1930. Worcester, MA: Clark University Press.

Watson, J. B. (1924). Psychology from the standpoint of a behaviorist (2nd ed.). New York: Macmillan.

Werner, H., & Kaplan, B. (1967). Symbol formation: An organistic- developmental approach to language and the expression of thought. New York: John Wiley.

Winter, D. D. (1987). Field studies of Action Profiling reliability. Movement studies, 2, pp. 21-22 (Published by the Laban/Bartenieff Institute of Movement Studies)

Winter, D. D. (1989). Somatic psychology: The contemporary and historical role of the body in psychological thought. Manuscript submitted for publication.

Winter, D. D. & Goldman, E. J. (1987, August). Molecular study of Action Profiling. Paper presented to the Action Profilers International Conference, Antwerp, Belgium.

Winter, D. D. & Schmickl, E. (1988, August). Concurrent validation of Action Profiling: Relationships with the Myers-Briggs. Paper presented to the Action Profilers International Conference, Toronto, Canada.

Winter, D. D., Widell, C., Truitt, G., Shields, T., & George-Falvey, J. (1989). Empirical studies of posture-gesture mergers. Journal of nonverbal behavior, 13 (4).

Wundt, W. (1973). The language of gestures. The Hague: Mouton (Original work published 1921).

Body-Mind Dancing™*

Martha Eddy, M.S., CMA

Introduction

To dance is to express what lies within, giving shape, form, and intensity to the inner intention of the mover. To dance, with or without the intent to perform, is to communicate, potentially addressing the full gamut of human experience. This communication may be intended only for one's own self-discovery, but the visibility inherent in movement implies the presence of an audience. Therefore, in all dance, even dance explored alone in a room, social behavior is implicit.

However, the purposeful cultivation of communal dance forms has waned as art has become secularized; the sacred aspect of art has dwindled across all the expressive disciplines (Moore, C. L., 1987). The major challenge for dance educators today is to re-embody a form of danced communion that speaks to all aspects of human experience. This parallels the challenge of re-training the public in the art of experiencing dance, since it is not well-appreciated (other than music-video dance and ballet) in comparison to the other arts. One way to raise public understanding of dance is to increase participation in dance classes. Dancing activates one's own bodily intelligence, enabling one to observe dance with greater responsiveness.

Dance teachers will continue to impart performance skills, such as the projection of personal energy from the stage to the audience. However, they should also be teaching body-mind communication, the embodiment of inner motivation, and the sheer pleasure of moving with others. They can also bring awareness to movement impulses, revealing the deep creative source that lies within everyone. Focusing on the emotion within the movement, rather than the outward appearance,

---

* Printed by permission of the author.

conveys the deep integrity of a truly embodied statement. Teaching dance from this perspective thereby becomes more appealing to both non-dancers and former dancers. This new approach to dance presents challenging goals for the dance teacher who wishes to develop more than physical proficiency.

New Insights into the Body-Mind

The feeling of movement can be taught kinesthetically. In the last twenty years, a burgeoning awareness of the body and its movement has taken place, so that dance pedagogy can now be a very different experience than ever before. This new understanding has been inspired by emerging sciences such as kinesiology, biomechanics, motor learning, sports psychology, athletic training, exercise physiology, and dance medicine. However, these analytic disciplines cannot supply the powerful emotions of awe and wonder, which are so necessary for artistic creation. Jungian and transpersonal psychological approaches are trying to re-integrate the traditional concept of the mind/body duality into a greater whole. The new somatic movement therapies (such as the Alexander Technique, Feldenkrais' Awareness through Movement, Bartenieff Fundamentals of Movement™, Rolfing, Skinner Releasing, Body-Mind Centering™, and Ideokinesis) have begun to bridge this internal and external reality.

Integration of the new body-mind perspectives from the sciences, body therapies and psychology has important implications for dance pedagogy. We now know, for instance, that learning through a variety of perceptual channels enhances retrieval of information from the cerebral cortex and accesses greater associative processes, especially when movement is involved (Rose, 1987). We know that mental imagery can improve movement skills, optimizing kinesthetically efficient movement (Sweigard, 1974), and can enable one side of the body to learn from the other (Feldenkrais, 1977). We know that non-verbal communication makes up about 60% of all human interaction, so we can use movement to improve communication skills (Moore, J., 1980). From the Eastern martial arts, we have learned that movement can increase self-integration, self-empowerment, and spirituality, and bring into conscious awareness the personal center from which movement impulses arise (Tohei, 1978). From advances in exercise physiology and biomechanics, we know how to increase blood flow to the muscles, increase the range of motion and optimize muscle strength to improve performance (McCardle, McCardle & Katch, 1981). As artist/educators, our task is to apply these advances to dance[1] particularly to modern and post-modern dance, as well as ballet (where this process has already begun). Both dancers and health professionals must keep in mind the dancer's challenge, to be "simultaneously athlete and interpretive artist" (Vincent, 1979, p. 2).

Body-Mind Movement Systems

Another important body-mind link originated in the work of Rudolf Laban, which was brought to the U. S. in the 1930's by Irmgard Bartenieff. This approach is now called Laban Movement Analysis (LMA). Laban's student, Warren Lamb, explains

> . . . the unique element which isolates Laban from his contemporaries in analogous fields is that although rooted in the study of body movement [his work] goes beyond the physical . . . . Laban saw movement as the common denominator of mind-body functioning which also takes in the spirit and expression of emotions (Moore, C. L., 1987, p. 10).

LMA teaches us the following universal movement principles (LMA Certification Curriculum, 1982):

1. All movement involves a constant interplay of mobilizing and stabilizing factors.

2. There is a need for recuperation after exertion; but this can be a dynamic change of energy use, rather than passive resting.

3. Dynamic energy shifts can involve changes in the body parts in use, spatial positioning, and exertion of weight, space, time and/or muscular tension.

4.   Movement occurs in all three spatial planes;
movement training ideally utilizes the complete
kinesphere (the area which can be reached without
taking a step).

Training in LMA includes the Space Harmony Scales,
geometrically proportional movement sequences that serve the
same purpose as musical scales (Laban, 1975), and the floor
and level-change exercises of Irmgard Bartenieff's
Fundamentals of Body Movement™ (Bartenieff, 1980).

Body-Mind Centering™ (BMC) is another holistic movement
system, involving thoughts and feelings expressed through the
body. BMC is an experiential approach to movement re-
education and analysis developed by occupational therapist
Bonnie Bainbridge Cohen, who also studied LMA. It is based on
anatomical, physiological, psychological and developmental
principles.

My lifelong integration of movement science, martial arts
(Aikido), body therapies, exercise physiology, kinesiology,
perceptual-motor development and Dance/Movement Therapy
led me to develop a new approach which I call Body-Mind
Dancing™.[2] Body-Mind Dancing™ is a system of movement
training that extends the principles of holism to the modern
dance classroom.

Body-Mind Dancing™ is influenced by my positive
experience with Dance/Movement Therapy, a process of
psychotherapy that uses dance or movement.
Dance/Movement Therapy provides sensitive listening to the
memory of muscles and the wisdom of the unconscious mind,
while paying close attention to transference relationships that
bring us in touch with aspects of our past that need healing.
Aside from the benefits of improving one's mental health, these
methods are also definite assets in choreography, personal
growth and in all aspects of bodily healing. Dance/Movement
Therapy, along with traditional verbal psychotherapy, can help
to address other psychological factors that affect dancers' lives.
Gestalt Therapy, Process-Oriented Therapy, Hakomi Therapy,
Bioenergetics, Co-Counseling and Psychosynthesis are other
therapeutic methods that include a strong bodily component.

Psychological concerns that have already been identified for professional dance company members include the pressures of hard work and low pay, constant travel with time and cultural changes, eating disorders, and body-image problems. Dance/Movement Therapy has the advantage of being a kinesthetic pathway to insight, which is often an effective avenue of self-discovery for dancers. Authentic Movement is a particular approach within Dance/Movement Therapy that is now offered in several dance departments and in summer dance festivals. It gives the mover an opportunity to spontaneously express movement impulses unbounded by preconceived frameworks and without pressure to achieve a particular outcome. This non-judgemental exchange is often extremely beneficial for relieving the emotional stresses of highly-trained dancers who have spent many hours of their lives having their movements dictated, controlled, reviewed, perfected, and judged.

Body-Mind Dancing™ draws particularly on the movement principles of LMA, BMC and the Kestenberg Movement Profile (KMP), developed by Judith Kestenberg. BMC, LMA and the KMP are externalized frameworks for understanding body movement, taught through a psychophysical training process. The Fall, 1990, course description of Antioch New England Graduate School lists the Body-Mind Dancing™ course as follows: "participants will return to rhythmic involvement in full-scale dance to enhance the embodiment of movement theories."

The Influence of the KMP

The KMP is related to LMA and BMC, because Kestenberg's early research was influenced by her studies with Irmgard Bartenieff and Warren Lamb. Several aspects of the KMP are similiar or identical to LMA, including the concepts of mobility and stability (Kestenberg & Buelte, 1983) and the framework of effort/shape (Dell, 1977). However, Kestenberg also adapted and expanded LMA in important new directions, especially as applied to the neurodevelopmental process of infants. The KMP has been particularly influential in providing detailed, in-depth psychological and functional meanings for a given type of movement and offering powerful research tools for human movement analysis. Some of Kestenberg's additions to movement analysis are:

1. Tension-flow rhythms and attributes.
2. Unipolar shape-flow and shape-flow design.
3. Precursors of effort (pre-efforts).

A comparison of the developmental perspectives of the KMP and BMC shows further contributions. Kestenberg provides a clear analysis of a child's progressive use of space. In the KMP, each of the first three years of life represents mastery of a new plane of motion (Kestenberg, 1975). She observed the first six years of childhood in great detail, leading to insights into adolescence and adulthood.

The KMP enhances the teaching of dance in many ways. It reveals richer detail for rhythm, movement patterns, group interactions and emotional expression. Dance sequences can be based directly on the KMP, or it can be used as a source for improvisation. KMP-based improvisations have subtle rhythms originating in developmental tension-flow patterns, such as sucking, biting, swallowing, etc. These tension-flow rhythms help clarify the emotional motivation behind physical movements. My students say that working with KMP imagery is emotionally involving, fun and meaningful, and stimulates the natural developmental flow of movement.

The KMP also sharpens the dance teacher's powers of observation. An understanding of pre-efforts helps me to see whether students are in a learning or defensive mode, and to recognise when they have mastered the rhythm and dynamics of a movement. For example, in teaching a highly dynamic movement involving a combination of efforts (such as strong, direct and accelerating), if instead I observe a flow-based movement (free or bound muscle tension) or a pre-effort-based movement (vehement, channeled or sudden), I might ask the student whether they are feeling successful or frustrated. Perhaps they need help to more clearly define the movement they are trying to learn. Using the KMP, I can develop activities to help students access their dynamic repertoire in an appropriate developmental progression. I am also able to perceive more about each student's feeling state by observing their habitual body shape and body attitude. These observations help me to assess variations in the mood of the group and the needs of individual class members.

In Body-Mind Dancing™, I use the KMP to describe rhythm changes, to increase the dynamic interplay of the class, and to observe shape changes for their choreographic content. I often use a developmental framework in structuring the flow of the class outline. I allow personal exploration time for expressing feelings and sensations (shape-flow activities), bridging and boundary-setting (arc and spoke-like movements), and finally planar and multi-dimensional relational activities (shaping in planes). This parallels the developmental progression of structuring self-feelings, defenses and learning modes, contacts with others and the cognitive creative process.

Another basic developmental framework is to proceed from floor activities to sitting, to standing, with careful attention to the transitions between those phases. The KMP inspires me to proceed from floorwork to standing with attention to the more simplified concept of planar use. This can become more complex by adding the reflex activities which are the baseline of both BMC and the KMP. Once the class is standing and moving across the floor, group movement can be allowed to emerge organically through attunement to a common rhythm: class members move through the room exploring different body movements to this rhythm (Kestenberg, 1975). Some of the emerging movement shapes are combined, and the group begins to mirror common shapes as well as the rhythm. The shared creative process leads to heightened appreciation and enjoyment of the resulting movement experience. Finally, the stretching activities that end the class include visualizing the organs beneath the stretched muscles. In terms of the KMP, this may involve tension-flow rhythms and shaping of space through all directions and planes.

The KMP also provides insight into one's style of teaching. For instance, I tend to teach in a containing rhythm, a mothering type of style. Kestenberg identifies this developmentally as a swaying (inner-genitally-derived) rhythm. This is the rhythm that a person (male or female) first experiences between ages three and four, while identifying with the mother's caretaking role and enjoying caretaking

(Kestenberg,1975). This rhythm has been successful for me, with mostly positive responses from students, such as "I've moved my whole body without ever feeling stress or competition."[3] However, it is beneficial for dance teachers to continually expand their rhythmic repertoire, to be able to teach a more lively and diverse class. The KMP provides a framework for this self-expansion.

Principles of Holistic Dance/Movement

Body-Mind Dancing™ is based on two universal human experiences: being in the body, and experiencing thoughts and feelings. It assumes an integral relationship between these two phenomena and seeks to bring them both into full awareness. It enables consciousness to be brought to various thoughts and feelings through the movement of the body. Therefore, while learning to better utilize our anatomical and physiological resources, we also learn to embrace our emotional and expressive selves, and this provides a powerful way to experience the mind-body connection. What better way to prepare oneself for creation or expression in an art form that requires the physicalization of thoughts and feelings?

Sondra Horton Fraleigh, dance philosopher and aestheticist, speaks to this view of dance as a physical art medium that resonates within the bodies of both the dancers and the audience:

> Because dance is in essence an embodied art, the body is the lived (experiential) ground of the dance aesthetic. Both dancer and audience experience dance through its lived attributes — its kinaesthetic and existential character. Dance is the art that intentionally isolates and reveals the aesthetic qualities of the human body-of-action and its vital life (1987, p. xiii).

While dancing from this body-mind union, our thoughts and feelings often emerge spontaneously, as different parts of the body express the messages of our different selves. Even when dancing spontaneously, patterns occur (as in all natural phenomena), as can be seen in the personal styles which permeate the works of most choreographers — whether their starting points were rational concepts or ineffable feelings.

BMC teaches that every part of the body and every physiological system has its own uniquely-patterned movement quality, and in some cases, spatial range, that we can consciously access. Cells are grouped by types of tissues: skeletal, muscular, nervous, organ, fluid and glandular. The first three types form the voluntary system and are the anatomical concepts most commonly explored in dance training. The remaining three systems are the areas in which we bring our awareness to the autonomic (involuntary) components of our body. Exploration of this subcortically controlled autonomic experience helps us to access unconscious feelings and information, and can assist us in our "journey toward wholeness" (Thompson, 1982, p. vii).

Laban was also interested in the nature of cellular existence, speculating that if we could follow the wisdom of individual cells, instead of the commands of complex governing units, we might learn from them both self-defense and self-sacrifice for the good of the whole: "all the possible virtues and volitions exist, and are fulfilled in an exemplary way, in the life of cells" (Thornton, 1971, 25). Of course, the wide prevalence of cancer and the growth of AIDS in our society show that even the cellular environment is not immune to damage and distortion and, in addition to its own cellular wisdom, needs to ally with what Laban calls the "central controlling mind" or "governing cell-groups" (Thornton, 1971, 26).

As one moves, one can change mood by varying the dynamics of spatial use, the level of physical exertion, or the locus of initiation. This allows one to experience different internal qualities that underlie different expressive statements, as taught in BMC classes. For instance, kicking the leg by activating the femur (thigh bone) and attending to the sensation in the iliofemoral joint (hip joint) is a skeletal image which brings out the intention of clarity. By placing one's attention on bones, the shape and form of the action becomes very precise and clear. Alternatively, one could perform the same kick while attending to the iliopsoas and other hip flexor muscles, bringing out more power and force, and perhaps a more assertive feeling. Or one could deepen the source of movement to the organic level by initiating the movement from the intestines. This would allow more obscured feelings to emerge, resulting in a more voluminous, three-dimensional action, possibly accompanied by an emotional association, such as letting go, surrendering or resisting. In this case the muscles and bones are still the primary movers, but the style and expression of the leg action is in-formed by a deeper organic intent. One could even allow the sciatic nerve to initiate the movement, adding an alertness and largeness to the movement: this nerve runs the length of the leg and stimulates its many sensory-motor choices. In each of these examples, all tissues of the leg are involved, with the musculo-skeletal system providing the primary force of locomotion. The difference between them is the mental intention that calls upon particular resources of the body, influencing the meaning of the action and eliciting, in the above cases, clarity, power, emotion, or alertness. At the same time, choosing to explore clarity, power, emotion or alertness through movements based on LMA or KMP could bring out these particular bodily resources, unless inhibited by deeply ingrained fear. The benefits of this approach to dance training are twofold: (a) ready access to a wide range of expressive potential, which is necessary to maintain the vitality of dance creativity, and (b) deeper awareness, understanding and nurturing of the body, since access to a variety of movement choices enhances body-mind health.

It is very important that dance professionals know the health hazards of rigorous dance training — including anorexia nervosa, bulimia, exercise-induced anemia, dysmenorrhea, amenorrhea, anxiety, and injuries to the musculo-skeletal system. These hazards can be greatly diminished by allowing students, dancers and teachers to take personal responsibility for their bodies and minds, since unfortunately the choreographer's artistic desires often defy the practicalities of both physical and psychological health (Vincent, 1979). This does not mean that professional organizations should ignore their dancers' health concerns, but rather should shift to a dancer-based approach. Bureaucracies adapt slowly, and dancers' own responses to training techniques, institutional conventions and the dance lifestyle/culture must be considered in order to keep the art of dance alive, healthy and up-to-date. Some commonplace dance practices may be forced to change for the better, if the participating dancers learn to trust their own experience and speak out about it. For dance to mature as an art form, dancers must be taught to carefully regard their own physiological and psychological experience. It may seem that there is no space or time in a dance class to learn the intricacies of physiology and psychology. How can one learn to dance while simultaneously attending to one's anatomy, physiology, kinesiology and emotional counterparts? The solution is a balanced attention to both the internal and the external environment, a major theme of both BMC and LMA. Healthy movement requires an integration of these two types of attention. Dance classes can teach this.

Movement/dance classes are available around the U.S. (and in Canada, Europe, Asia and Australia) led by teachers trained in BMC, LMA, KMP or other somatic education systems.[4] In these classes, which utilize knowledge from somatic movement, this balanced use of inner and outer concentration is a conscious objective. New names are often created for these approaches, since their experience offers a different level of awareness and sensitivity than traditional dance classes. This new approach to teaching dance, with all its variations, quite possibly will be fully absorbed into the mainstream of dance technique training (including ballet). Although the end result — a holistically trained dancer — is potentially magnificent, a word of caution is in order about this process: the shift from the present paradigm can be disruptive, especially if introduced haphazardly or forced in an untimely way. Our present training paradigms, based on the ethics of elitism (with its struggle for competition and petty individualism), challenge a dancer's technical prowess only, and in making the shift to empowering the whole person by training their body-mind, we are asking dancers and teachers for a major change of consciousness.

Teachers may speculate that this shift would produce more choreographers than ensemble dancers. If the holistic training is complete, however, dancers will actually appreciate both self-initiated expression and participation in group dances created by others. Holistic training could also minimize the addictive and co-dependent behavior that is now rampant among dancers, fostered by the super-authoritarian approach to teaching dance technique. This approach dictates not only the dancer's attire, attitudes and demeanor, but exactly where to position what parts of the body in space, and to what rhythm, in accord with the dynamics of the movement style being taught. Closed skill sports and choreographed dances leave little room for personal expression. Ideally, performers could select the movement style which matches their creative and expressive needs. Often this does not happen, however, especially with child dancers.

Application of Holistic Principles

Holistic learning, involving experiential anatomy, kinesiology, and physiology, can occur in the context of a dance class. I use the following six-phase class structure, loosely based on a traditional model of a modern dance technique class (class format can vary from week to week or even day to day and class length can vary from 50 minutes to three hours):

Phase I: Information about anatomy, kinesiology, and/or physiology.

Phase II: Warm-up.

Phase III: Floor exercises (includes partner work for kinesthetic and tactile learning aides).

Phase IV: Center floor and across the floor full-out moving.

Phase V: Further synthesis of anatomical information into dance (long dance sequence, solo or group improvisational structure).

Phase VI: Cool-down and stretch-out, including non-verbal and verbal sharing about the experience; questions and comments.

Outline of a lesson plan

The objective of this class is to learn the musculo-skeletal kinesiology of the ilio-femoral joint within the context of a dance class.

Phase I of the class begins with pictures or skeletal parts that depict the active interaction between the ilium and the femur in an iliofemoral flexion. In Phase I we might also work with partners, in either a quadrupedal or side-lying position, to locate bony landmarks (greater trocanters, ischial tuberosities, etc.) which are potential points of initiation of movement. Attention could be given to isolating this action from spinal flexion and extension, as leg work is often performed with over-involvement of the back. Different movements would then be explored, with the femur as either the active mover or the stable support (leg swings or pelvic extensions). These movements readily lead to an improvisational warm-up (Phase II), beginning with self-attunement. This leads into Phase III by gradually increasing the circulatory rate with an exercise sequence of leg swings and pelvic extension/flexions, done on the floor. Phase IV includes a standing variation, while focusing on maintaining the clarity of action that was achieved with the partner's help in Phase I. This could lead into Phase V, a long dance sequence that involves battements, jumps, and moments of balancing on one leg, followed by turns initiated by a twist of the pelvis. This choice of actions exhibits a periodic alternation of proximally and distally initiated ilio-femoral movement. Phase VI, the cool-down, would most definitely include a thorough stretching out of the hamstring and quadricep muscles as they often tighten (and strengthen) considerably in classes that include repeated ilio-femoral action.

Discussion might include a review of those principles that enhance a balanced use of muscles around the ilio-femoral joint (proximal-distal alternation, use of rotation, etc.) and comments about the state of mind elicited by working in a concentrated way with this joint and the muscles surrounding it. (Although during each phase after Phase I, every other major body part is also brought into active movement.) This focus on the ilio-femoral joint might lead to responses such as feelings of power, centered connectedness, and the ability to move through space more effectively.

Analysis of a Lesson Plan

The following section explains the logic of each phase of the class, while giving more in-depth examples of teaching about the autonomic as well as the musculo-skeletal functioning of the body.

Phase I teaches some aspect of anatomy and physiology, using a particular part of the body. This will include how that body area affects movement when focused attention allows its particular quality of expression and non-verbal message to emerge. Experimenting with these images in class, it is helpful to take them to their exaggerated limits, focusing on one part of the body-mind, for the sake of clarity. For instance, imagine doing a progressive spinal roll-down from a standing position by passively allowing your bones to drop into gravity, one at a time. Now imagine this same action done by actively lengthening the muscles of the back (eccentric contraction) and then using the same muscles with shortening (concentric) contraction to rise back up. These two experiences have very different dynamics and states of mind. Letting the bones fall with the pull of gravity is a very passive state, allowing the laws of nature to exert more control than usual. Moving by fully contracting the musculature is a very active doing, which may be accompanied by feelings of power, vitality and strength. Intense muscular initiation is done less in dance than it is done in sports, so the quality of the movement appears as athletic dancing.

Phase II begins with enough low-intensity aerobic activity to get the blood circulating to even the deepest musculature. In Body-Mind Dancing™, class often begins with this warm-up process, in the form of a structured improvisation to help students get in touch with their specific body needs on that particular day. Specificity is an important principle of sports training that is also needed in dance: in a form of movement which uses thousands of different body actions, an individual's idiosyncratic movement patterns and life habits need to be taken into account in preparing to move, even in the most predictable and stylized actions. To satisfy this need, the Body-Mind Dancing™ improvisational warm-up includes both a physiological component (aerobics, circulation) and a psychological component (self-attunement). This can come, for example, from smooth level changes from the floor to a standing position, and back down again, with a conscious awareness of breathing rhythms. These movements can be accompanied by images such as "feeling supported by the floor," "bonding with the earth," or "befriending the pull of gravity" to increase stability. Other warm-up methods could include:

(1) large shifts in weight (varied stepping patterns), finding one's own rhythm and then interacting with others;

(2) vigorous whole-body swinging, emphasizing release of control, followed by suspended lightness and the resulting feelings.

The student personalizes each of these warm-ups, selecting their preferred use of movement intensity, body parts, pace and spatial configuration. Actively watching, the teacher monitors further for safety and effective warm-up.

Movement that is relatively formless, such as shaking and wiggling, can facilitate a gentle circulating effect of the synovial joint fluid and the blood. In these movements, the body fluids may be used as the primary initiators. Although muscle action causes the movement to occur in space, the subtle coordination and quality of the shaking movement is governed by the reality of moving the body fluids, increasing the circulatory flow. Again, the body-mind statement being made is that of willingness to loosen up. Often students will be shy to shake in this way until they feel that the rest of the group is actively involved and non-judgemental about the silly playfulness that results from letting go of muscular control.

It may be difficult to fathom the concept of using conscious movement of body fluids to spark a sense of freedom. However, physicists know that all matter moves. The mind-body link shows us that in every externally-visible movement, there is an invisible cellular response, and that each movement that stimulates a particular pattern of cellular action is associated with a specific point of view or attitude. As humans have

observed each other through the ages, we have at times sharpened and at other times neglected our ability to perceive another's mood, personality characteristics, or state of health from non-verbal cues. So if you don't usually jiggle or shake in your dance warm-ups, you may be surprised by the benefits that can be derived from it. For instance, for a person with
• arthritis or bursitis, the image of jiggling the synovial joint fluid can be used as a metaphor for achieving greater fluidity and a greater range of body-mind movement.

During Phase III, which includes floor and level change exercises, it is often appropriate to reinforce experiences from ontogenetic (childhood) movement history that help babies develop balance and locomotor abilities. For instance, the explorations of the ilio-femoral joint described earlier can be related to neurodevelopmental movement skills, such as pushing homologously or homolaterally, crawling, creeping and standing up (Cohen, 1984, 1989; Batson, 1987, p. 13).[5] Continuing in Phase III, the teacher may choose to take either of the themes from Phases I or II (skeletal initiation versus conscious muscular initiation, or the active use of body fluids) to create a series of floor or level change sequences that further exemplify these energetic contrasts, perhaps focusing now on the dynamic results of alternating them.

In Phase IV, the class moves into even more vigorous, large-scale activities, and can play with different rhythms as the foundation of the movement impulse. For example, the class could follow the rhythm of the arterial pulse, with faster shifts of weight or with rhythmic jumping — like aerobic dance. Or they could experiment further with body fluids, using the rhythm of the venous blood returning to the heart, perhaps in large waltz-like swinging motions. Since venous circulation is not assisted by the muscular action of the heart, it can be helpful to assist the return of the venous blood with squeezing movements of the fingers and toes, using the distal body parts as a peripheral pumping mechanism. For those with a blocked heart function, the "venous" rhythm provides a more gentle approach than the "all out" arterial rhythm. The teacher can either present these movement sequences, without elaborating on their effects (perhaps in a conventional modern dance technique class) — or the teacher can describe their physiological basis. The decision whether or not to explain the underlying rationale and effects of the movements should be made with the overall continuity of the class in mind.

These experiential visualizations can also be seen and interpreted by a viewer. Sometimes the viewer can clearly distinguish these shifts of quality or mind, and sometimes they cannot be perceived at all. Whether as mover or viewer, however, one does not need to consciously know all about physiology and the psyche in order to experience the dance; anatomical systems and their dynamics are used spontaneously, because they are inherent in the movement itself. One can inspire the same body-mind experience by motivating movement with descriptors from the KMP or LMA, such as **light**, **strong**, **bound**, **free**, **direct**, **indirect**, **accelerating** or **decelerating**. A full variety of expression results from our intention to express the full diversity of our selves, including all of our body parts.

In Phase V, the intent is to dance, to feel the full joy of moving, and perhaps to prepare for performance. At this time, the teacher can let go of the physiological information, allowing it to become the background knowledge that helps the student develop a new skill. Or, the teacher can guide the entire class in freely experiencing anatomical imagery through a structured improvisation. For example, different dancers could choose different biological rhythms (arterial, venous, lymphatic, cerebro-spinal, cellular breath exchange, etc.) and then interact with these diverse rhythms (as a whole or in half groups), imagining that they are one body, with the room as the skin, the outermost membrane.

Awareness of Our Movement Repertoire

There are times when we strive to broaden our movement range to get out of a rut, to communicate better, or to learn and accurately perform the style of a particular teacher or choreographer. The use of the KMP, BMC, and LMA to structure the elements of movement and their meanings allows us much greater access to diversity of expression.

We also benefit by gaining greater awareness of the very tool that we use to create our art, like a visual artist learning the difference between pastels, guache, oils and watercolor.

Movement artists benefit from information about different body tissues, a dynamic resource to bring greater health and balance to the body. Stress develops in the body when the same actions are done repeatedly: after a while, the mechanisms in use become physically and emotionally worn, stuck in a fixed behavior pattern. When this happens, we can ask ourselves what we need; what part of ourself is dormant, unexpressed, repressed; what aspects of ourselves do we need to express, to feel as whole? Since stress can also result from the need for adaptation when the organism perceives that it is already in homeostasis (Seelye, 1974), a case can be made that an expanded dynamic repertoire, with its broader definition of homeostasis, reduces stress by giving us greater flexibility to cope with change in our inevitably changing lives (Bartenieff, 1980).

I use my skeletal leverage/articulation and the sensitivity of my nervous system as unconscious themes in my movement repertoire. I do hands-on body work in which I use the receptors of my nervous system to assess another's condition, and then act with clear structure and leverage to present new options. Therefore, it is helpful for me to actively express my feelings (from my organs) and my intuitiveness and rhythmicity (from my glandular system) in my movement choices during the day, rather than be guided by neuro-skeletal control at all times. This also leads to taking care of the body; being aware of the potential for injury prevention, while simultaneously increasing expressive range.

I'm very excited about the power of sharing the feelings stimulated by dancing (in Phase VI), whether through singing, talking, questioning, or fully expressive dancing. By being open to this interchange, especially during the cool-down phase (when it won't disturb the developing momentum), it's amazing how smooth and well-integrated the class remains. This opportunity to exchange also breaks the traditional pattern that technique classes are the teacher's stage, rather than the students' laboratory.

After participating in the class, students are often curious about some significant aspect of themselves that they have never considered before, or excited about a new sense of their bodies (for instance, their spine feels longer). I have had many students tell me that their self-image has changed, or that their perceptive ability has been enhanced. What they are describing is movement re-patterning created by metaphorically meaningful movement sequences and hands-on contact. This re-patterning occurs because information, in the form of imagery, about our basic structural existence is being processed. Furthermore, we are activating an exertion-recovery cycle that allows the body enough time to rest, and even heal after over-exertion.

Summary and Conclusions

It is both artistically and physiologically useful for a dancer to understand anatomical principles: how to warm up by activating body fluids, how joints work most efficiently, how to fully activate the muscles, and even how to integrate the functions of organs and glands to add greater volume to movement. As we explore these concepts, the result is both increased range of expression and ease within the body, created from mental shifts accompanied by an easy, relaxed parasympathetic state.[6]

Potential teachers of this integration of dance science and psychology-in-action need to become familiar with the flexible format of such classes, which distinguishes them from typical modern dance classes. For instance, in Body-Mind Dancing™, each class involves improvisation, vocalization, hands-on work and anatomical discussion, as well as movement sequences. In order to properly teach Body-Mind Dancing™, one needs to be an experienced dancer who is certified in either KMP, BMC or LMA, with additional training in their application to dance teaching. The potential teacher also must be comfortable working with students at different levels of skill since people with a wide range of dance ability are attracted to this approach and I encourage it. In Body-Mind Dancing™, mutual respect grows out of the shared vulnerability of the participants, who learn from each other as well as from the teacher (modeled after Aikido). This highly valuable exchange follows the holistic paradigm of the body-mind connection by emphasizing horizontal relationships versus vertical (hierarchical) relationships in the dance classroom. It goes hand-in-hand with focusing on our personal reasons for studying dance, so that we are not distracted by self-judgement and inappropriate competitiveness. There are other benefits to class diversity: at times all class participants are able to share their reactions with each other; and, a person who lacks training in dance, but has a background in other areas, often has a fresh outlook on movement, inspiring even a highly-skilled professional dancer. That can be terrifically insightful, especially when the performer is attempting to communicate to an audience of non-dancers. Working with this dynamic mixture of people is extremely rewarding.

On occasion, however, it is helpful to separate groups by skill level, in order to appropriately challenge balance, visual-motor memory, range of motion, and strength for each student. So far, the skill level of Body-Mind Dancing™ has been primarily at the level of the intermediate dancer, so new dancers have not been put into potentially injurious situations. In any case, advanced dancers can always benefit from a slower class, especially when the focus is on making new physical connections, which requires concentration by everyone. It is interesting that many dancers who have suffered injuries have re-entered dance through Body-Mind Dancing. ™

Another aspect of this training that balances differing levels of dance movement ability is the use of the neuro-developmental framework. We are all on an equal level when exploring our developmental roots. This includes activities such as discovering our responsivity to stimuli which elicited primitive reflexes in infancy, righting reactions (that upright the head), and equilibrium responses (off-vertical balancing). In pure activities such as the neuro-developmental movements of rolling, creeping, crawling, sitting up, standing and walking, everyone has areas of potential improvement; everyone has some aspect of perceptual-motor ability that can be enhanced (an underlying premise of the KMP, BMC and Bartenieff Fundamentals of Movement™).

The teacher of Body-Mind Dancing™ also benefits from some training in dance therapy or some other psycho-therapeutic method, in order to appropriately handle the emotional reactions resulting from body exploration that will occur in the classroom and to perceive and maintain boundaries. The training received in somatic movement therapy (inclusive of Bartenieff Fundamentals and Body-Mind Centering) aims to improve physical functioning and in turn enhance expressivity and a person's overall sense of well-being. Dance/Movement Therapy achieves this end-result also, but through a psychodynamic interaction requiring several years of training. For instance, classes on the heart can bring out strong emotions of pain and sadness. Deep feelings can become fixed in our body tissues, remaining there until they are unlocked by physical expression, movement or vocalization. After these feelings are expressed — whether experientially through movement, or outwardly through verbalization to others — people often feel a greater sense of camaraderie, joy and lightness, which is reflected in their dance.

The teacher's responsibility is to provide a safe environment for this exploration. However, the teacher must also convey the message that the class is an educational setting, not a therapy group, and maintain this boundary. When psychological issues regarding a person's past or present arise, it is wise to have a dance therapist to refer them to.

Each discipline benefits from an understanding of the other. Medicine provides excellent diagnostic information. Physical therapy unfolds a wide gamut of manual techniques and kinesiological principles that many dancers need to be aware of in their work. Somatic movement therapy brings knowledge of physical illness and wellness and how to embody avenues for cellular healing. Together they make a strong team. A dance class that integrates as much of what is current from science, somatics and psychology becomes an active vehicle for meeting dance's most basic purposes: eliciting the satisfaction of outwardly expressing that which lives within, that which words cannot always explain; activating bodily resources in such a way as to increase one's life force; working with the body fully enough to have a good night's sleep; sharing with others in rhythmic harmonies and common feelings; and playing.

Intensified group bonding, increased interpersonal interaction, and rediscovery of personal experience inform dance, bringing it alive and imparting "real" meaning to technical prowess.[7] It is inspiring that a process which improves dance technique also leads to a keener awareness of the richness of human experience, and that from this awareness also follows the re-emergence of the sacred aspect of dance. The re-discovery of the sacred aspect of life on earth has been a valuable contribution to our world in the 1980's and 1990's. With this incentive it becomes truly joyous to be dancing into the twenty-first century!

References

Bartenieff, I. (1980). Body movement: Coping with the environment. New York: Gordon & Breach.

Bartenieff, I. & Davis, M. (1965). Effort/shape analysis of movement: The unity of expression and function. New York: Dance Notation Bureau Press.

Batson, G. (Fall, 1987). Balancing stability with mobility for dynamic spine function, Part III: strengthening the trunk. In Kenneth Laws & Ann McNeil (Eds.). Kinesiology for dance, 10 (Special issue), 12-16.

Cohen, B. B. (1982, Spring/Summer). The training problems of the dancer. Contact Quarterly, 9-15.

Cohen, B. B. (1984, Spring/Summer). Perceiving in Action. Contact Quarterly, 24-39.

Cohen, B. B. (1989, Spring/Summer). The Alphabet of Movement, Part I. Contact Quarterly, 20-38.

Cohen, B. B. (1989, Fall/Winter). The Alphabet of Movement, Part II. Contact Quarterly, 23-38.

Dell, C. (1977). A primer for movement description using effort/shape and supplementary concepts. New York: Dance Notation Bureau Press.

Eddy, M. (1991). Past beginnings. Movement News, 16, 14-16. (Published by The Laban Institute.)

Feldenkrais, M. (1977). Awareness through movement. New York: Harper & Row.

Fraleigh, S. H. (1987). Dance and the lived body. Pittsburgh: University of Pittsburgh Press.

Kavner, R. (1985). Your child's vision: A parent's guide to seeing, growing, and developing. New York: Simon & Schuster.

Kavner, R. & Dusky, L. (1974). <u>Total vision</u>. New York: Simon & Schuster.

Kestenberg, J. S. (1975). <u>Children and parents</u>. New York: Jason Aronson.

Kestenberg, J. S. & Buelte, A. (1983). Prevention, infant therapy and the treatment of adults. III: Periods of vulnerability in transition from stability to mobility and vice versa. In J. Call, E. Galenson and R. Tyson, (Eds.), <u>Frontiers of infant psychiatry</u>. New York: Basic Books.

Kestenberg, J. S. & Sossin, K. M. (1979). <u>The role of movement patterns in development: Vol. 2</u>. New York: Dance Notation Bureau Press.

Laban, R. (1975). L. Ullmann (Ed.), <u>The language of movement: a guidebook to choreutics</u>. Boston: Plays.

McCardle, W., McCardle, F. I., & Katch, V. L. (1981). <u>Exercise physiology: Energy, nutrition, and human performance</u>. Philadelphia: Lea & Febiger.

Moore, C. L. (1987). The Laban lecture: Beyond words. <u>Movement and dance</u>, 76, 7-14. (Published by The Laban Guild, Surrey, England.)

Moore, J. (1969). <u>Neuroanatomy simplified</u>. Dubuque, IA: Kendall Hunt.

Moore, J. (1980). <u>Neurobehavioral sciences and their relationship to rehabilitation</u> (videotape series). Rockville, MD: American Occupational Therapy Association.

Rock, J. & Mealy, N. (1988). <u>Performer as priest and prophet</u>. New York: Harper & Row.

Rose, C. (1987). <u>Accelerated learning</u>. New York: Dell Trade Books.

Tohei, S. (1978). <u>Ki in daily life</u>. Tokyo: Ki No Kenkyukai.

Scarry, E. (1985). <u>The body in pain</u>. New York: Oxford University Press.

Seelye, H. (1974). <u>Stress without distress</u>. Philadelphia: Lippincott.

Sweigard, L. (1974). <u>Human movement potential: Its ideokinetic facilitation</u>. New York: Harper and Row.

Thompson, H. (1982). <u>Journey toward wholeness: A Jungian model of adult spiritual growth</u>. New York: Paulist Press.

Thornton , S. (1971). <u>Laban's theory of movement: A new perspective</u>. London: Plays.

Vincent, L. M. (1979). <u>Competing with the sylph: Dancers and the pursuit of the ideal body form</u>. St. Louis: Andrews & McMeel.

Notes

[1] See <u>Kinesiology for Dance, Vol.10</u>, #1, Sept. 1987, for an extensive bibliography of books on Dance Science.

[2] The author has an M. A. in Exercise Physiology (Columbia University), is a certified Laban Movement Analyst and Certified Teacher of BMC, also holding certifications in Massage Therapy (AMTA) and Holistic Health Education (Eugene and Eva Graf). She worked in behavioral optometry as an intern with Richard Kavner. She has taught for eight years on the Certification faculties of the School for Body-Mind Centering and the Laban Institute of Movement Studies. She has been on the faculty of the graduate dance therapy departments of New York University (1984-1988) and Antioch New England Graduate School (1989-1992) and various other dance department faculties. She co-led dance therapy workshops with Ute Lang. She is currently acting president of the Laban Institute of Movement Studies. Besides teaching, she loves to choreograph and perform.

[3] This caretaking rhythm has broad implications in a culture that has been predominantly based on masculine values. The male or female mover who recognises the basic human need to nurture rediscovers traditionally "feminine" qualities, which have been profoundly undervalued. This increases their understanding and integration of the Yin polarity — the unconscious, intuitive feminine wisdom — increasing respect for the arts, which necessarily arise out of these creative depths. This enhanced sensitivity also supports the spiritual aspect of dance; while dancers often experience a form of rapture (even in a traditional technique class), contemplation of the spiritual aspect of the creative process has usually been neglected. Body-Mind Dancing™ gives movers the chance to rediscover and commune with the divine seed of their inner creative process (using certain quiet rhythms,

Authentic Movement, etc.).

4 A partial list of universities teaching holistic movement classes: University of Washington; University of Texas, Austin; St. Olaf College; Hampshire College; Antioch New England Graduate School; Connecticut College; Hope College.

5 Note that there is an error of terminology in Batson's article, as she describes two different neurological body part organizations by synonyms: ipsilateral and homolateral. In BMC, the term "homologous" is used to describe movements initiated and performed with bilateral symmetry.

6 Other articles could easily be written on topics such as body-mind approaches to injury prevention, improved protocols for balancing anaerobic and cardiovascular endurance training in dance, and the physiological ramifications of a low percentage of body fat (refer to Bainbridge Cohen, in Contact Quarterly, Spring/Summer 1982, and Fitt in Kinesiology for Dance.

7 "'Real' meaning" is used here in the sense of W. H. Auden's use of real in describing the plight of the modern day poet, as compared to those of the past: "The real meant 'sacred' or 'numinous.' A real person was not a personality but someone playing a sacred role, apart from which he or she might be nobody (Moore, 1987, p. 8)." Real in this sense includes the spiritual as well as the material.

Acknowledgements

The author wishes to thank Liz Aaronsohn, Kathie McCarthy, Liz Paddy, Ruth Pollock and Paul Feuerstein for editorial comments, Susan Loman for her support, and Irmgard Bartenieff and Bonnie Bainbridge Cohen for their inspiration.